WHO COUNT AS PERSONS?
Human Identity and the Ethics of Killing

WHO COUNT AS PERSONS?

Human Identity and the Ethics of Killing

JOHN F. KAVANAUGH, S.J.

GEORGETOWN UNIVERSITY PRESS / WASHINGTON, D.C.

Georgetown University Press, Washington, D.C.
© 2001 by Georgetown University Press. All rights reserved.
Printed in the United States of America

10 9 8 7 6 5 4 3 2 1   2001

This volume is printed on acid-free, offset book paper.

Library of Congress Cataloging-in-Publication Data

Kavanaugh, John F.
    Who count as persons? : human identity and the ethics of killing /
by John F. Kavanaugh.
        p. cm. – (Moral traditions and moral arguments)
    Includes bibliographical references and index.
    ISBN 0-87840-836-3 (alk. paper)
        1. Life and death, Power over. 2. Philosophical anthropology. I. Title.
II. Moral traditions & moral arguments.

BJ1469 .K38 2001
179.7–dc21   00-061018

To brothers and sisters at the margins—
of society, of economy, of health

The traditional ethic is still defended by bishops and conservative bioethicists who speak in reverent tones about the intrinsic value of all human life, irrespective of its nature or quality. But, like the new clothes worn by the emperor, these solemn phrases seem true and substantial only while we are intimidated into uncritically accepting that all human life has some special dignity or worth. . . . Hardly anyone really believes that all human life is of equal worth.

PETER SINGER, *Rethinking Life And Death*

Was it wisdom Mao Tse-tung attained when—like Ted Bundy, who defended himself by pointing out that there are "so many people"—he awakened to the long view?

"China has many people," Mao told Nehru in 1954. "The atom bomb is nothing to be afraid of. . . . The death of ten or twenty million people is nothing to be afraid of." A witness said Nehru showed shock. Later, speaking in Moscow, Mao displayed yet more generosity: He boasted that he was "willing to lose 300 million people"—then, in 1957, half of China's population.

An English journalist, observing the Sisters of Charity in Calcutta, reasoned: "Either Life is always and in all circumstances sacred, or intrinsically of no account; it is inconceivable that it should be in some cases the one, and in some the other."

ANNIE DILLARD, *For the Time Being*

Contents

Preface

An early draft of this work began with the words, "This book begins in Zimbabwe." The words are no longer in the present text because so much time has passed. Yet I still owe to my African students there the confirmed belief that philosophical encounters with life and death are crucial to our world and our common humanity. They had no texts, almost no personal books. They did, however, have a desire to investigate just what makes us human persons—and they were willing to pursue the ethical implications, even if they required a painful change of mind.

Since those years in the 1980s, I have made many more formal presentations of the labors presented herein. I have received, as well, ample assistance and challenge in offering my ideas, although I am sure I cannot remember everyone who gave me assistance and warning over the years.

I presented general notions of the assault on personhood and the theory of endowed personal nature at Marquette University's Center for Ethics Studies; the Center published "Recovery of Personhood: An Ethics After Post-Modernism" as a monograph in 1995. I presented an early formulation of my theory of value at Notre Dame University at a conference that was published as *The Challenge of Global Stewardship*. My contribution—"Intrinsic Value, Persons, and Stewardship"—finds echoes in part of Chapter 5 of this book. In reviews that I have written—usually on books that treated consciousness, human nature, and ethics—for the *Modern Schoolman*, as well as observations in *America* magazine's "Ethics Notebook," I have developed ideas that appear herein, even to the extent of some shared central terminology.

In presentations to medical students and the philosophy department of Creighton University; in a year as McKeever Chair at Saint John's University and faculty member at Saint John's CHAP program for hospital administrators; in presentations at Milltown Park in Dublin, Ireland, and to the Jesuits of South Africa; and during a wonderful tenure as visiting scholar at the Hastings Center, I was able to offer many of my judgments and evidences for friendly challenge and wise advice. Finally, parts of Chapter 8 were presented in a keynote address, "Healing the Person," to the Catholic Health Association National Assembly in June 2000.

In addition to the two blind readers of my manuscript (who offered thorough, honest, and critical evaluations—even though I'm sure they disagreed with my position), I am indebted to readings by Jeff Puttoff, S.J.; Mark Chmiel; Ellen Rehg; Garth Hallet, S.J. (who saved me from the more outrageous characterizations of consequentialism); William Rehg, S.J.; Patrick Murray; Jeanne Schuler; Joseph Drew Callahan, M.D.; Vallee Willman, M.D.; and Danielle Darriet, M.D. I think I can honestly say that none of them fully agrees with all of my arguments; as was the case in discussions with Eleonore Stump; Walter Ong, S.J.; Teka Childress of the Catholic Worker; and Donald Merrifield, S.J. however, I always came away from the encounters more thoughtful, careful, and meditative. Philip Fischer, S.J. was helpful with the editing.

My undergraduate students in medical ethics at Saint Louis University and the participants in a philosophy seminar on Aquinas and natural law (including Kevin Decker, who helped me organize my bibliography) have showed me how profoundly difficult it is to propose the theory I offer. Finally, Mellon grants enabled me to study at the Hastings Center and, for a week in July 1999, to observe and collaborate with Danielle Darriet, M.D., at Helio-Marin in Berck-sur-Mer, France.

Although I have not given much of my labor to men and women in distress, my greatest thanks go to those who work and live at the margins of human life. They live at L'Arche communities in India, the house of the dying in Calcutta, the Catholic Worker community in Saint Louis, and the nursing homes and extended-care facilities in Zimbabwe and France, as well as the United States. I also have been challenged by people who supported and suffered violence in Africa, Ireland, India, Latin America, and the United States.

JOHN KAVANAUGH, S.J.
SAINT LOUIS UNIVERSITY

1
Introduction

"Person" signifies what is noblest in the whole of nature.
Thomas Aquinas[1]

Philosophy springs from human persons. All philosophies must. Even those that deny our personhood are—like it or not—posed by actual human persons making the denial.

Thus, this book is situated in the tradition that understands philosophy as a centuries-long discourse about the truth of our humanity. What kind of beings are we? What are we to do? Unlike some contemporary approaches in philosophy, this book is not based on the conviction that such questions should be repressed or ignored.[2] Instead, it is based on the certitude that there would not be any philosophy—or, for that matter, any human enterprise—if there were not beings like us, capable of self-knowledge in relation to the world. Ultimately, our personally reflective engagement with our own lives is the secret of philosophy's attraction and power. Philosophy, no matter what its form, is of and about humans. It is not merely about the "idea" of humanity. It is about us: living actual persons. We are the hidden topic of every philosophical conversation.

The fact that *we* are the issue is preeminently clear in ethics. At least, that is the point this book makes. Two claims are at the heart of its effort: One, that human personhood is the foundation of ethics and two, that if we desire to *do* ethics, we cannot repress or negate the very personhood that drives us to do ethics in the first place. In some ways, these claims are ancient, and efforts like this one have been made before. In other ways, however, the claims are profoundly new; in our own day, many people have concluded that there are neither foundations for ethics nor any rationally compelling arguments for moral convictions. Regarding the claim that ethics requires an implicit affirmation of personal dignity, we live in a world in which men and women, young and old, are increasingly considered worthless—whether in Bosnia, Lebanon, Cambodia, Rwanda, or American streets and hospitals.

Like generations before us, we are confronted with two basic ethical questions: What does it mean to be a human person? Are those who count as human persons suitable candidates for killing? These questions invite a dual investigation. The first task is to develop a philosophical anthropology, or what might be referred to in other quarters as a philosophy of human nature or a philosophy of mind. The second task is to show how such a philosophy of the person leads to and grounds an ethical system and provides a framework for answering what I will propose is the foundational but preeminently practical ethical question: Is it ever morally permissible to intentionally kill a human being?

There are many difficulties accompanying the task of this book—not the least of which is the vast range of material written on every issue it addresses. "Nature," "person," "self," and "mind" are topics to which entire libraries are devoted. There is even a considerable bibliography of documents relating to the proposition that such terms are meaningless. Yet we must examine these notions if we are to do the kind of ethics we propose.

Likewise, the specific topics of killing—physician-assisted suicide, abortion, euthanasia, terrorism, and capital punishment—already have volumes devoted to them. Each topic, moreover, is hotly contested by antagonists speaking out of different histories and often employing different vocabularies.

Although I take note of such antagonists, histories, and lexicons in this book, I do not examine them in depth. Offering even one coherent ethical theory is weighty enough. Let this work be inspected for what it is: one approach—a minority and radical approach, in the contemporary context—to the phenomenon of persons in the world.

In human behavior, however, much more than mere theory is at stake: Living, breathing persons are. From Tel Aviv to Somalia, from Baghdad to Los Angeles, from Liberia to Haiti, arguments over human rights and human dignity are not settled in seminar classrooms or scholarly books. They are settled through starvation, with missiles, at the muzzle of a gun. In every part of the world, I have heard the defense of terrorism from right wing and left wing. In every part of the world, humans are *theoretically* held in highest esteem and assumed to have great dignity, claiming impressive rights that are appropriate to that dignity. Yet in every part of the world, in the name of a relentlessly ubiquitous "realism"—under the guise of race, class, quality of life, sex, property, nationalism, privilege, security, religion, or ideology—men and women are willing to wipe out men and women. Today, any human being is a candidate for elimination, from someone's perspective. The tactic takes one of two forms: Either exclude such humans from our definition of meaningful or "full" personhood or, if forced to accept them as persons, justify the killing of them in the name of a greater good or more pressing value.

One could wonder (perhaps too apocalyptically) whether this new century will be the era of personhood extinguished. More immediately and practically, I argue that the repression and even the degradation of personal life already extend into every segment of our private, interpersonal, social-political, and theoretical worlds. Such depersonalization is "dialectical"—that is, it is an organic phenomenon that cuts across our entire life-world. It is a dynamic process whereby presumably separate areas of our lives actually interpenetrate in an organic system of experience.

We cannot neatly separate the "private" world from the "political" or "cultural" world. The erosion of family and neighborliness, for example, is as much an economic phenomenon as a civic and personal experience. Likewise, these personal and civic realities are expressed in and are expressions of our "theoretical" or "academic" world. In our philosophy and literature departments, we relate to each other economically, interpersonally, and professionally. There is a politics and a theoretics of privacy. There is an economics of academia and interiority. If we ignore the dignity of personal life in these areas of our experience, we should not be surprised that claims of personhood are repressed in war, penal systems, and hospitals.

Our personal lives are not insulated boxes. They are mirrors of cultural ideology, practical instances of high theory, and vulnerable membranes permeated by the consumer society's life-blood.

Thus, any attempt to recover and "reconstruct" or "recenter" the person in ethics must be systemic. It must cut across every area of our lives. We must see how the recovery of our personhood cannot be simply an ethical issue or an academic problem: It is a lived task, worked out in every realm of our consciousness—as professionals, as scholars, as laborers, as parents or spouses, as social activists, as political agents, as people of faith. It will be dialectical.

The recovery and reaffirmation of human personhood cannot be accomplished by academic work alone. It will not be achieved through mere theoretical analysis or some isolated instance of personal illumination or any political program. All of these human arenas interpenetrate. They receive their very legitimization and power by their mutually supportive relationship to each other. Academic life is a function of the market and the entertainment media; politics is a function of amusement and cultural distraction; the project of living one's "private" life is subject to the benefits as well as the perils of advanced industrial capitalism and technology.

As a work of philosophy, this book surely is meant to engage students who investigate the foundations and implications of ethics, not only as a theory but as a vital concern that touches their private and civic lives. It also is meant for their teachers—to some extent as fellow professionals and specialists but more fundamentally as persons. For it is our shared personhood that unites all teachers and students. Thus, this book is for anyone who wants to investigate just what it might mean to be a person—and whether it makes any difference.

What readers will find here is an interpretation of the ways that personal reality is devalued and a proposal regarding ways it may be recovered. This work is neither a book of readings nor an historical survey. Its purpose is to formulate a view of the human person that embraces our animal existence as well as our personal endowments; establish a theory of intrinsic value, not only of every species but preeminently of the personalized human species; integrate an objective ethical system with our identity as ethical animals; and defend the extremely controversial position that intentionally killing a human person is never ethically permissible.

If these goals are met, they will challenge many of the approved opinions of our culture, our academic world, and some of our strongest private preferences. They also will carry disconcerting implications about the way we should live and die. The final proposals—that an authentic ethical life requires the habits of interiority, intimacy, and openness to "marginal" persons—might even appear "unreal" to us in the context of this culture and what it deems the "real" world. Yet this feeling of estrangement, I believe, itself depends on *what* is most "real" to us, *why* it seems so "real," and who informed us about its contents.

Our ordinary lives, which are shaped in so many ways by our cul- •
ture's economic relationships, media system, and social dynamics, are
lived out in the context of an unquestioned and—by that very fact—
controlling "reality system." The "real" world that we appeal to as a last
court of judgment is a world that has its own criteria of reliable knowledge, its own metaphysics (what is most real and substantial to us), its
own religious philosophy (what is worth living and dying for and what
gives us ultimate meaning). Obviously, it has its own ethical system as
well. Notions such as "value," "worth," importance," and "quality of life"
are not spun out of our heads or taught exclusively by parents and
schools. They are social, cultural, and economic constructions.

Over the past 25 years of teaching university students, I have come
to realize that confusion in ethical discourse is related to the fact that
there are presumed "reality principles" underlying certain unquestioned
economic, political, and cultural myths. Many of these principles—for
the most part unnamed—inherently conflict with any ethics that affirms
the irreplaceable value of the human person. People may *want* to believe
in the intrinsic dignity of human persons—and even act courageously on
that desire—yet they seem unable to muster any rational defense for
their beliefs or desires. The programming of cultural ideology relativizes
all convictions about the worth of a human being. The value of persons
over property, the worth of a personal life despite its woundedness, the
sacredness of the human body, and the privileged place of humans in the
world all seem terribly unreal amid the clamor of money, media, and
politics.

The dominant North American culture, moreover, affirms Utilitarian dogmas of "use value," happiness maximization, and almost uncon-
strained liberty in anything except property rights. To suggest that
there are values other than utility, that happiness may be no guarantee
of ethical integrity, and that the limits of liberty are constrained by the
dignity of the being who bears liberty is not merely counter-cultural. It
actually seems unreal.

I also address that "real world" in this book. I examine how ethical
issues of life and death are inextricably tied to cultural propaganda. I
also propose that, if we take seriously what being a human person
means, we must resist much of what seems to be required for acceptance
in the "real world."

This book is written in solidarity with academicians who think that
realities such as persons, killings, bodies, culture, and human vulnerabil-

ity are prime candidates for philosophical reflection. It also is motivated by the conviction that ethics, grounded in a philosophy of the person, is crucial if we are ever to understand or justify moral passion—whether Bertrand Russell's, Mohandas Gandhi's, or one's own.

Some professional philosophers will not sympathize with the approach or conclusions of this effort. I entertain the hope, however, that the issues might at least be engaged or that teachers of philosophy might with their students investigate a formulation of human dignity such as this—if only to refute it. Some readers may even be further encouraged to continue their efforts to personalize their lives or recenter humanity at the table of philosophical discourse with fuller, more elegant, more compelling argument and analysis. Many philosophers and ethicists are developing strong responses to problems that this study only approaches and suggests.[3] Others have offered measured critique of the premises and convictions upon which this ethical approach is built. Endnotes, often with more specialized commentary, honor these facts. The central thrust of this project, however, is directed to one goal: the grounding of moral discourse in the reality of human persons, without whom there could be neither discourse nor morality.

Although the discussion in the pages that follow is in some ways academic and technical, I have written to address our ordinary lives. I try to communicate in a language that is not overly abstract, in a way that makes sense. I do not mean that sustained argument can be bypassed or that strange terminology is not used. I do mean, however, that I have made every effort to connect ethics to common experience. After all, that is where we live. If ethics has no impact on life, if it doesn't help us interpret our world or guide our action in it, it will have little worth.

What, after all, are the philosophical foundations of the moral outrage that we all experience when a child is terrorized or tortured? Richard Rorty has written, "When the secret police come, when the torturers violate the innocent, there is nothing to be said to them of the form: 'There is something within you that you are betraying.'"[4]

My position is that Rorty is incorrect. Indeed, there is nothing we might say to terrorists that *forces* them to change their minds. Yet this acknowledgment does not mean that we cannot *say* it to them. In fact, we *ought* to say it to them—and know *why* we say it. We must understand *why* such viciousness is a violation of the moral order itself, and why we are correct in taking measures to prevent it.

Thus, the rest of the project opens before us.

In Chapter 2 I examine the ways in which human persons are systematically depersonalized in their private lives, in their relationships, in the social order, and in the discipline of philosophy itself. This reflection is meant to show the dialectically related and mutually supportive patterns of life and thought that prompt us to negate the personhood of our own lives as well as others. The themes of Chapter 2 are echoed in Chapter 8, where I propose patterns of personal recovery and reintegration.

In Chapter 3 I examine just what being a person—as a living, bodied being—means. Accepting our bodies, in their vulnerability and ambiguity, as inextricably part of our identities helps us understand that we are neither efficiently functioning brains nor pure consciousnesses but animals that are uniquely endowed with self-expressive powers.

In Chapter 4 I propose that, as a natural species, we are capacitated from our very beginnings with inherent, yet-to-be realized physical and nonphysical endowments. Chapter 4, together with Chapter 3, attempts to answer questions about what makes us human persons and who should be included in such a category. These two chapters serve as a philosophical foundation for the claims I make in subsequent chapters that developing or damaged humans are indeed persons and deserve to be treated as such.

In Chapter 5 I investigate some characteristics of the ethical world that emerge from personal animals, the varying attitudes that people take when they enter moral reflection and discourse. I argue that ethics is a matter not only of internal dispositions and motives or external consequences but intrinsic values as well.

In Chapter 6 I characterize the ethical world as having the same multidimensionality that human persons do. Moral judgment—the very meaning of conscience—occurs only because persons are endowed with such a capacity. Although conscience is primary in moral decision and choice, it is as fallible as the humanity by which it is made possible. It also is as subject to challenge. The preeminently challengeable (and incorrect) judgment of conscience, I hold, is the acceptability of intentionally killing persons.

Chapter 7 is, in many ways, the crucial stage of my reflections. I initially apply the ethical prohibition against intentional killing of persons to self-defense and terrorism. I then bring that prohibition to bear on the medical issues of physician-assisted suicide and the termination of what are sometimes called "marginal" human beings. I not only contest the notion of "marginality"; I also reject the acceptability of intending to kill any human. An important contention is that intentional kill-ing is not a "premoral" phenomenon, like unintended killing, nor is it murder, as it is often understood legally, pertaining to malicious motive.

In Chapter 8 I return to the theme of dialectical integration. The recovery and fostering of personal life is achieved not only in the partic-ular prudence of ethical decision. It is won by integrating personal life-disciplines—engaged in solitude, encountered in intimacy, and ex-pressed in human solidarity, not only with one's intimate relationships but with every human, even the most wounded and marginal. I hope that such "disciplines" of the personal form of life will foster men and women to be less inclined to will the direct extinction of human life.

The epigraphs at the beginning of this book present starkly con-trasting assessments of the human situation. In *For the Time Being*— a tragic-poetic encounter with human suffering and history—Annie Dillard raises (after a painful inventory of disability, maiming, mayhem, and horrific loss) the possibility that every mother's child is either in-trinsically sacred or of no worth at all. This alternative suggests itself when Dillard contemplates Mao Tse-tung's willingness to coolly sacri-fice 300 million Chinese in a nuclear exchange. Mao's ruthlessness is only one instance of human sacrifice on the altar of history and human contingency—with its litany of brain-damaged neonates; profoundly handicapped, forgotten victims of tidal waves; the broken and the dis-eased. Dillard hints that our hunger for meaning and transcendence points to a human dignity that is more basic than any transient achieve-ment or desired goal.[5]

Peter Singer, an internationally prominent writer about ethics, has room for neither the transcendent nor the sacredness of human life. In an early passage of *Rethinking Life and Death*, Singer announces, "I do not speak in hushed tones when I refer to the traditional ethic of the sanc-tity of human life."[6] He proposes, instead, that our moral worth lies not in the kind of beings we are but in the activities we are capable of per-forming. Thus, for Singer, many and possibly all functioning animals carry greater moral weight for us than marginal humans who perform miserably and incompetently.

Although I have not constructed this book as a refutation of Singer, I do propose an account of the human person that opposes all "performance" theories of personhood. Moreover, I argue that the de-nial of intrinsic human dignity undercuts ethics itself. Such an effort need not require "reverent tones" or episcopal status. In fact, as a philosophical effort, the arguments and interpretations I offer do not rest on any religious commitment—although men and women of faith might find rational confirmation of their beliefs.[7]

I propose that the splitting of our personal existence from our human and animal reality is a dualism of Cartesian proportions. Indeed, not all persons are necessarily human. Yet all humans are persons—animals of special endowments that separate and valorize them above all other living organisms on this planet. "Marginal" human persons, who appear in many arguments about animal rights as well as human infanticide and euthanasia, are just that: marginal humans; they are members—albeit damaged, undeveloped, or rendered incompetent—of our personal community who not only require our respect but reveal our own vulnerability.

Thus, I have dedicated this volume to them, our brothers and sisters, those included in the class of beings that Thomas Aquinas has called the noblest in nature.

2

Personal Losses

Repeat. Do you read? Do you read? Are you in trouble? How did you get into trouble? If you are in trouble, have you sought help? If you did, did help come? If it did, did you accept it? Are you out of trouble? What is the character of your consciousness? Are you conscious? Do you have a self? Do you know who you are? Do you love? Do you know how to love? Are you loved? Do you hate? Do you read me? Repeat. Come back. Come back. Come back.

Walker Percy
Lost in the Cosmos[1]

One man who knows Trump well does see a rhyme and reason. Trump is a brilliant dealmaker with almost no sense of his own emotions or his own thoughts, this man says. He is a kind of black hole in space, which cannot be filled no matter what Trump does.

Time *magazine*[2]
January 1989

There are two unities to be explained: the unity of consciousness at any time, and the unity of a whole life. These two unities cannot be explained by claiming that different experiences are had by the same person. These unities must be explained by describing the relations between these many experiences, and their relations to this person's brain. And we can refer to these experiences, and fully describe the relations between them, without claiming that these experiences are had by a person.

    Personal identity is not what matters.

Derek Parfit
Reasons and Persons[3]

TRACES OF LOST PERSONS

In *Lost in the Cosmos* (subtitled "The Last Self-Help Book"), novelist Walker Percy portrays a world of robbed personhood in American thought and culture. The final passage of the book, supposedly addressed to us earthlings by an unnamed extraterrestrial being, is a press of questions—a catalogue of the moral inquiry that we have somehow suppressed.

Percy believes that the "Lost Self" occurred when American society and its institutions gave up vital convictions about our own humanity. We sacrificed these convictions in the name of a freedom to be endlessly entertained and indulged. Yet the freedom paradoxically masks a tyranny that exacts from us the tribute of our interior lives and authentic identity as persons.

Spread before us is a stunning repertoire of scientific and technological expertise; we need only exploit them for the enhancement of our "selves." Such selves, however, seem elusive at best, distasteful at worst. We have either lost touch with or actually rejected the selves we are so intent on fulfilling.

The only "selves" available to us are amnesic, bored, empty, ungrounded, escapist, sated, and in constant dread of being found out. Through it all, Percy is puzzled that we are so devoted to the quest of finding out whether chimps or extraterrestrials might communicate with us while we are strangely incapable of communicating with each other.

Our weekly iconographers—*People*, *US*, or *Time* magazine—provide cultural commentary on the emptiness in media stars' lives; these celebrities shine before our adoring faces as having "made it," although they have lost everything else. The supreme achiever, endlessly advertised in the life of someone such as Donald Trump, is little more than a "black hole in space." We find the paradox not only in our amusements but in our politics. The most successful presidential campaign may well be the one that has been most adept at concealing the identity of the person who hides under carefully constructed images.

In this chapter, I point to reflections in our private, cultural, and academic worlds to suggest how a diminished image of the personal self is mirrored in all three. In other words, philosophical accounts of "human identity" are just as thin as our media portraits and just as externalized as our own self-understanding.

Philosopher Derek Parfit's claim, after 200 pages of *Reasons and Persons*, that "personal identity is not what matters" reflects the problematic nature of our cultural and interpersonal lives. Although his technical book is a serious and painstaking work, often elegant in argument and crisp in style, it is bereft of any sense of personal, lived experience. He is most comfortable and reassured with thought experiments—machine metaphors, transmitter fantasies, and other possible experiences that a disembodied human might have. The living, breathing, ordinary self-conscious person is not there. In this considerable work—which has received and will continue to receive much commentary from the philosophical world—there is no sense of human teleology, no sense of any substantial personal identity, no presence of passion or desire. Such possibilities seem not to arise for the author.

Parfit's quandary is that he is incapable of imagining a human self that is anything other than a mechanical brain or a disembodied Cartesian ego. Parfit is not alone. Many philosophical treatments of human existence condemn us to a schizoid choice that we persons are either airy, insubstantial ("ahistorical" is a favorite word) "selves" that can be literally "nowhere," or highly localizable bio-computers, either reluctantly or eagerly identified as brains. The "self" is either a ghost (no thing) or a machine (no self). Obviously, with such constrictive alternatives, the self has to be lost in the philosopher's cosmos as much as it is in the social-political galaxy.[4]

Whatever happened to real people in philosophy? As the passionate Miguel Unamuno once complained, "The individual human, this flesh-and-blood human, is both the subject and supreme object of all philosophy, whether certain self-styled philosophers like it or not."[5] Claims that Unamuno was misinformed do not make it so.

We cannot out-jump our shadow. We cannot undertake any journey—philosophical or otherwise—from any place other than where we stand as conscious of ourselves in history. Unamuno's point is inescapable. The origin of all quests and questioning, philosophical or otherwise, is the living human person. The inquiring self—even if it cannot be discovered through meticulous analysis or reductive explanation—is the place from which every human effort, including philosophy, must begin. There would be no ethics if there were no human persons asking themselves questions about their identity, their purpose, and the import of their actions. Nor could there be any theoretical or practical science.

As Percy suggests, however, our perplexity is that the very question of human identity that underlies all secondary human questions is the one we seem farthest from answering—or even asking. The flesh and blood human that strangely disappears in fragmented private and social worlds also is banished from much of contemporary philosophical discourse. Percy's mourning of the lost self applies to scholarly journals as much as it does to mass culture.

A few philosophers believe that this situation is for the best. They advise that questions about meaning and human destiny should be abandoned. Indeed, some thinkers recommend that questions of human identity, if not totally inaccessible, should be relegated to fields of endeavor that are not properly considered philosophical. Richard Rorty, who is probably the most "famous" philosopher in the United States, proposes that the preeminently personal search for "answers" to questions about our meaning and destiny be given up by young and old alike. "The hope that one of them will do just that [find an answer] is the impulse which, in our present culture, drives the youth to read their way through libraries, cranks to claim that they have found The Secret that makes all things plain, and sound scientists and scholars, toward the end of their lives, to hope that their work has 'philosophical implications' and 'universal human significance.' In a post-Philosophical culture, some other hope would drive us to read through the libraries and to add new volumes to the ones we found."[6] As for trusting our immediate ordinary experience, neuro-philosophers such as Patricia Churchland propose that such matters be relegated to "folk psychology" as we move on to formulate a more sound, scientific philosophy that has no need of selves and personal interior lives.[7]

Thus, we find that logical, linguistic, formal, historical, or computational enterprises are called philosophical, while terrain leading to the most urgent moral quests is traveled more frequently in literature, psychology, and even medicine. Psychologist Rollo May undertook the great task of investigating the experience of human creativity and freedom. Psychiatrist Bruno Bettelheim dared to raise the question of "man's soul." Walter Ong probed the meaning of the self, but as a literary critic of astounding originality. Oliver Sacks delves into the mystery of personhood—but he does so as a neurologist.[8]

Yet the great integrative question of all philosophy that Kant proposed—"What is the human?"—is rare in contemporary academic philosophy.

We experience ourselves as driven to seek out our truth, yet so often we repress and dampen the drive itself. We hunger to be free of delusions, yet we continually entertain them.

This conflict between the repression and liberation of our person-hood ranges throughout our personal, social, and theoretical worlds. To find and accept the true self or to flee it: This dilemma is a constant oscillation in our experience, even if we are not given the title of philosophers. It assaults us in personal crises, pushes and pulls us through our relationships, and hounds our political conflicts.

Our interior world, our interpersonal world, and the world of ideas interpenetrate. We can never fully segregate any of these realms from the others. Yet we can at least focus on them one at a time, in reflection and conversation, well aware that no part of life is lived in isolation. Because any question always must begin as one's own, let us attend to the questions of personhood we experience in our interior lives.

THE FEAR AND CALL OF PERSONAL REALITY

The question of personal meaning inhabits every moment of true solitude and accountability. We encounter it the instant we recognize pretense in our lives. We face it as we glimpse the chasm between our public appearance and our interior actuality.

"Looking good is everything." So we construct our external looks according to the dictates of fashion and acceptability. Yet we are confounded in those rare times of recognition when we are actually little known and consequently little loved. Sudden acknowledgments that we live in fear of "being found out" alternate with dread of having never been truly known. We feel it when we realize how much we are fakes.

In *The Fall*, Albert Camus portrays our tendency to deceive as almost a vortex which sucks us into deeper and deeper turns as we relentlessly elude being named or known. Far more than any philosophical treatise, this monological novel unmasks our ruses and our ploys. The confessional tone of Jean Baptiste Clamence is almost seductive as it slowly pulls us into a confrontation with our own interior fraudulence and our avoidance of self-revelation.

I navigate skillfully, multiplying distinctions and digressions, too—in short I adapt my words to my listener and lead him to go one better. . . . With all that I construct a portrait which is the image of all and of no one. A mask, in short, rather like those carnival masks which are both lifelike and stylized, so that they make people say: "Why, surely I've met him!" When the portrait is finished, as it is this evening, I show it with great sorrow: "This, alas, is what I am!"[9]

Camus uses this seemingly honest self-revelation to trigger our own manifestation of conscience—if we dare.

Every experience of our fraudulence—as well as every slight intimation of our authenticity—prompts questions concerning who and what we might be. We are drawn into the most intimate of inquiries: What is most enduring and significant in life? Are we expendable and of little consequence? What are we really worth? Does anything last? Do we? Is there anything we do that endures?

Questions hound us with nagging reminders of our sheer contingency: the sadness of acknowledging that we are not necessary to the world or others, the pain of fleeting temporality, the shock of sudden death or blind destruction, the passing of years and friends, the changing of passionate concerns, the quick urgencies that we may try to drug out of consciousness or escape with distraction.

Ecstasies, too, prompt questions. We find ourselves suddenly stunned in the presence of beauty, awestruck at the utter vulnerability of birth or love, rapt in the splendor of music or thrilled by a brilliant athletic performance. In the truth of utter solitude, in the ebbing of any ecstasy, if we allow it, we cannot *not* ask: Who am I? What am I to do?

These experiences of our private world are mirrored in our interpersonal lives. The question of personhood is not posed in some isolated cocoon. We cannot even encounter ourselves outside of relationship. The mutuality of being known and knowing, of being loved and loving, is intrinsic to our history. It is central to our existence—whether we complain, with Jean Paul Sartre, that hell is other people or delight, with Martin Buber, that all real living is meeting.

An old Shona blind man in a hut near the Zambesi murmured to a young visitor: "If no one visits to see me, I will no longer be anyone." The question of the "I," though uniquely my own, finds its expression and answer in relationship.

When we allow ourselves to settle deeply into the experience of being in relation with another, we unavoidably face, once again, the questions at the core of our being. A man experiences the terror of being unimaginably frail and vulnerable in the presence of another person; a woman discovers a hidden interior rage unleashed by hitherto unknown forces of passion or fear. They ask themselves: Rather than entertain the pain of these questions, is it safest not to love at all?

Questions spill out from us when we are shattered by the ache of being loved, the frustrations of love's disappointments, and the bittersweet delights of its consummations.

Commitments rise up before us as terrors. Then, sometimes they flower as promises of finally being free. In some moments we bridle at being defined by others—so much so that our whole being resists. We want to be wanted, hunger for the familiar, find comfort in the expected. Yet expectations, rules, roles, and cultural programming jam our possibilities and seem to suffocate our hopes.

You and I are never really conscious of this world of persons without a trail of questions stalking us. What is it about myself that makes me so? What is it about our longings that they so easily deplete us? What abiding truth is there to our loves that soars and aspires to permanence? Do our choices and behaviors count? Why are the actions of another person like myself so revelatory of a power I never encounter in the world of objects? Why do you threaten me in a way I have never experienced in the presence of even the loveliest of animals? Why is there so much at stake for myself in my own actions? And why am I offended when my actions are taken away from me?

True, cultural concoctions and artifacts can repress the surge of questioning sprung from solitude and intimacy. As Mark Crispin Miller has written incisively in "Big Brother is You, Watching," Orwell's fantasy of the emaciated and tamed self is dangerously close to actuality in a consumer media-culture that trumpets, "We shall squeeze you empty, and then we shall fill you with ourselves."[10] Christopher Lasch has searched our new consumerist world where the self is, paradoxically, both narcissistic and minimal.[11]

Our cultural information system often reads like a catalogue of the wounded self: "Young People's Suicides: Epidemic," legitimized euthanasia, extended drug use, the crazed complaining phantasmagoria of talk shows, the dreadful fear of violation while we live in deadly fascination with it, and an almost narcotic use of television.[12]

The wound of the self is the wound between selves. Commitments wane and, incomprehensibly, dissolve. Communities, civic and familial, tremble. Intimacies are as thin and rare as the philosophical theories that might treat them. The very bonding of interpersonal steadfastness that might reengage, reveal, and confirm our personal value is too frail to bear the task. Cultural institutions seem able to offer only escape from the pain of personal encounter, with one's self or with others. Despite all the satisfactions of our consumer culture, an underlying personal dissatisfaction remains. The mighty *Forbes* magazine celebrated its 75th year in a 550-page issue with the cover story, "Why we feel so bad, when we have it so good."[13]

Notwithstanding our flight from ourselves, the very avoidance of personal and interpersonal encounter serves only as a constant reminder of the threat from which we flee: entering the personal realm in oneself or in the other and avoiding the answers such encounters require of us.

SOCIAL AND POLITICAL DEPERSONALIZATION

The inescapable questions that mark our rare moments of solitude and inhabit our rarer moments of true intimacy are the same questions that, on a grand scale, haunt our social, political, and cultural worlds. The same puzzling maze of human value, personal dignity, and individual significance is woven into the fabric of claims concerning rights and justice. The tattered whole unravels, however, in a constant pull of paradox. With haphazard logic, persons are alternately degraded and exalted.

Proxy wars are manufactured, billion-dollar jets are constructed, and scenarios of devastation are objects of research and development. Peoples of the earth are willing to mount deadly arsenals to adjudicate competing claims over human destiny; they are willing to see children scalded in the name of these same claims; they are willing to sacrifice the future for them.

Where do these claims come from? Every child knows enough to ask why. How do we know what we claim about humans? What evidence do we give to support it?

Minorities, women's groups, gay rights groups, animal rights movements all demand that just treatment and respect be paid. Yet there is an astounding absence of any corporate sense about what the foundation of rights may be, other than a covert appeal to self-interest and power—themselves, the very motives and values used to justify the action of the purported oppressor.

When an underling of the Ayatollah Khomeini called for a retaliation ratio of 5 to 1 against Americans, a hue and cry over such barbaric morality was heard from the newspapers of the United States. Yet only a few years before, a conservative American columnist had suggested that President Ronald Reagan make a speech ending with the words: "In the future, and on principle, we guarantee that we will retaliate for the death or injury of any U.S. citizen at the rate of 500 to 1. As I speak to you, I have received word that 15 Shiite villages and their inhabitants no longer exist."[14]

The disregard for human life that roams the streets and generates feckless "commissions of concern" is weirdly confirmed by the 18,000 murders in 22,000 hours of television watching that the average high school student has seen by graduation day. All rhetoric of concern and compassion is refuted by the realities of 15 million starvation deaths every year and one-quarter of the world's population living in chronic malnutrition. The romantic imagery of the loved child is rebuked by the facts that homicide is one of the five leading causes of death in early childhood in the United States and that this country has the second-highest childhood homicide rate in the world. The myth of the cherished child is rebuked not only by babies in trash cans but by state-legitimized infanticide.[15]

We hear constant appeals for justice and human dignity in China or Serbia, in the urban ghetto or the U.S. Congress, in the pubs of Northern Ireland or the opinion columns of social commentators. What is it all about? Is this moral urgency merely a function of fashion, supply and demand, and class interest? Or is there some intrinsic human value bestowed upon every human person regardless of state pronouncements or media interpretations?

Is the human person expendable? Why, or why not? Or when? And for what reason may I consider you expendable—or more expendable than others?

In the Court TV of popular opinion, what prevails in most appeals to human dignity is a self-interest that divests others of that very appeal on familial, national, racial, or sexual grounds. Thus, the terminally ill, "the enemy," the "scum" on death row, the unwanted, the families of terrorists, or those of a different class are rendered expendable. In every case a self-contradictory logic, based on values exalted as absolute, is used to render them expendable.

I have met the IRA operative who saw only hypocrisy in Margaret Thatcher defending England's "just war" against Argentina on the very principles she was unwilling to allow to the IRA. Thatcher's "inviolable rights" worth dying and killing for were not, it seemed to him, a function of our humanity but a function of being British.

A Palestinian knows quite well that the State of Israel was founded with the help of the same acts of "terrorism" that it condemns before the world—this, while thousands of innocent Arab children suffer violence and poverty at the hands of "legitimate authority." Muammar al-Qaddafi knows the two-facedness of a country that is outraged by the murder of an American hostage while it is tolerant of three hundred Lebanese being destroyed in a bombing. He knows the deception of a leader who condemns the manufacture of chemical war instruments while his own country is not only manufacturing such instruments but has also amassed devastating nuclear stockpiles for the sake of its national security. A Sandinista knows the contradictions of a church leader who vividly condemns the violence of a revolutionary movement—while the same leader gingerly tiptoes around the fact that powerful Christian nations rely wholeheartedly on the power of munitions to secure their securities. A Kurd or an Ethiopian knows that there is more than moral principle involved, more than "concern for humanity," when Kuwait is liberated but their own bondage is ignored. In the face of such contradictions, it becomes quite clear that, whereas the dignity of the human person is the first principle to which we appeal, it also is the first principle to fall.

Guadalupe Carney, a chaplain for a revolutionary force in Honduras, put it simply before he was killed in his Central American hills: "You capitalists say that we should not support a revolutionary army because it advocates violence as a means of conflict-resolution. And yet you do the same for the most powerful army in the world. What is your principle: Only big armies are morally acceptable? What do you think we are, fools? Are we not human too?"[16]

Carney, like so many others who experience or identify with victimhood, saw that our moralisms are little more than a hodge-podge of principle appealed to and evaded. People make the pretense of morality in the very act of violating it. For the cleverest among us, the showmanship of emotional moralizing accompanies the most hard-hearted neglect of the poor. Regardless of the political or media pretense, conscience is compromised.

Basic moral logic and sensitivity are under siege. That siege, again, forces the questions: *Why* do we make claims for human dignity? And why do we *suppress* them so easily? Why is there moral outrage? And why is it so selective? What is it about us humans that, when violated, moves us to moral condemnation?

Behind all of these quandaries are the most basic of ethical questions: Who count as human persons? And when may we legitimately eliminate them?

The task of our ethical investigation is to find an answer to the question of persons and their expendability. This task will require us to search out the conditions that make human questioning possible and to pursue the implications in our findings.

IMPERSONAL THEORY, DE-PERSONED PHILOSOPHY

Certainly a major task of philosophical ethics is to determine just what human persons are and then to examine the implications of destroying or degrading them. Rarely, however, does the academic world confront such issues—despite all the interest in the "self" or "the mind-body problem" it seemingly promotes.

In a remarkable and honest exchange with protesting German students during the 1960s, Herbert Marcuse touched on the core issue underlying all claims to resistance in the name of justice: an objective moral law grounded in the dignity of the human person.

> The doctrine of the right of resistance has always asserted that appealing to the right of resistance is an appeal to a higher law, which has universal validity, that is, which goes beyond the self-defined right and privilege of a particular group. And there really is a close connection between the right of resistance and natural law. Now you will say that such a universal law simply does not exist. I believe that it does exist. Today we no longer call it natural law. But I believe that if we say today that what justifies us in resisting the system is more than the relative interest of a specific group and more than something that we ourselves have defined, we can demonstrate this. If we appeal to humanity's right to peace, to humanity's right to abolish exploitation and oppression, we are not talking about

self-defined, special group interests, but rather and in fact interests demonstrable as universal rights. That is why we can and should lay claim today to the right of resistance as more than a relative right.[17]

Marcuse was issuing a double challenge. To those who would resist social change, he appealed to intrinsic human rights, in the name of which such changes are demanded. To social activists who would demand social change, he insisted that such a demand is groundless and ineffective if there are no such intrinsic rights to appeal to.

Marcuse might well have issued the same challenge to the academic world. Whether under the standard of natural law, human dignity, or the inherent value of a human self, every issue of justice and morality is an issue of the person. Just as actual, breathing persons are undergoing an interior struggle of disintegration versus affirmation and are witnessing a social struggle of ennoblement versus degradation, so too in the academic world there is a constant conflict of approach and avoidance with respect to the human person.

In more dramatic and daring cases, it appears as if post-Heideggerians, postmoderns, post-structuralists and pragmatists, deconstructionists and anti-theorists all have mounted a rostrum to proclaim the "end of man" or the end of humanism or the end of the self or the death of the soul. Behind much of this talk is the disenfranchisement of the human person.[18]

Even Alasdair MacIntyre's attempts to ground ethics in virtue theory and rational discourse have been marked, until recently, by a strange absence of the *subject* of ethics, the one who *does* ethics: the person. *After Virtue*, which appeared 10 years after John Rawls' breakthrough *Theory of Justice* (which itself contained no sustained discussion of the inherent endowments of the moral agent and their relationship to rights), was marked by a pessimism over the chaos of moral discourse and the loss of foundations. MacIntyre turned to custom and tradition—the very solution that Marcuse in the 1960s understood was inadequate in the face of competing cultural relativities—rather than the human person. Thus, the answer to *Whose Justice? Which Rationality?* was not "the person's" but that of competing cultures and traditions, no one of which could claim superiority over any other. "There is no standing ground, no place for enquiry, no way to engage in the practices of advancing, evaluating, and rejecting reasoned argument apart from that which is provided by some particular tradition or other."[19]

MacIntyre's efforts to explore the social and cultural contexts of moral belief and practice surely were an antidote to any pretense that ethics could somehow be worked out independent of context and tradition. He also demonstrated how some traditions are more inclusive and capacious than others. Yet he neither provided nor called for a discussion about the human subject, that particular kind of being in the world that is somehow *capable* of producing both traditions and moral life. To be sure, a human cannot "stand" anywhere but in a particular place and time. What makes all the difference, however, is what kind of being is doing the standing.

For example, the thirteenth chapter of *Whose Justice? Which Rationality?* appeared to have been misnamed. MacIntyre entitled it "The Rationality of Traditions." Yet how can there be any tradition without living persons to build, sustain, and communicate it? Might his chapter not better have been titled "The Rationality of Persons" or "The Humanness of Tradition"?

Such questions may well be behind MacIntyre's latest move away from a somewhat disembodied or purely cultural or tradition-based account of ethics and human reality. Although *Dependent Rational Animals* is still an investigation of virtues and cultural forces, it breaks open (as the title suggests) the powerful implications of the fact that we humans are indeed animals with special capacities.[20]

MacIntyre's philosophical journey suggests an alternative to the dominant accounts of the human person as ghost, machine, or "ghost in the machine." It is an embodied, self-conscious animal life. Let us admit: It is a blessing that the grand claims about some timeless and spaceless "autonomous man" have been unmasked as fraudulent strategies that justify power and self-interest. Yet not every possible model of the human person is a pretense. Nor is every theory of humanness based on outrageous claims about persons utterly disengaged from history and space.

What if there is a notion of the person that never entertained Cartesian or Kantian delusions of grandeur in the first place? More important, what if there is an embodied, substantial, and historical agency called the human person who builds, is fed by, and transforms all traditions, as well as languages and philosophies? This question merits attention.

Human beings, by virtue of the way they are constituted, by virtue of their endowments and capacities, bring something to every culture and all conversation. We may not be separable from our historical and social contexts, but we are not reducible to them.[21]

Just as you cannot have culture or agriculture without agents who have sown them, you cannot have language without the speaker, interpretation without the interpreter, or communication theory without the communicator, community of communicators, and theorists.

The remainder of our task is to investigate just what kind of being the human being is and to examine what humans uniquely introduce to the world. This investigation joins the ranks of a growing number of philosophers who are tracking down traces of the human person within culture, language, art, and nature. Indeed, such investigation is found in the phenomenological, personalist, and Thomist traditions.[22] It also appears, I believe, in the writings of Jurgen Habermas—who continually is called upon to defend himself against the dogmatic charge of creeping humanistic "foundationalism." At his best, he is guilty.[23]

Richard Bernstein's *The New Constellation* is one of the strongest reminders that philosophy ultimately is about persons. Bernstein points out that even Michel Foucault, so relentless a debunker of core human identity and foundational values, has to covertly appeal to some notion of value and some notion of human agency. Maybe humans do not have some "hidden" essence, but Foucault nonetheless appeals to the fact that humans somehow are the "kind" of beings that can marvelously invent, reproduce, and project themselves. Bernstein unmasks the double bind that Foucault imposes in *requiring* the very things he has forbidden us to do—to find out what a personal self is. Thus Bernstein: "What is perhaps most ironical about Foucault's talk of ethics and freedom—as it pertains to our historical situation—is that its intelligibility presupposes the notion of an ethical or moral agent that can be free and that can 'master' itself."[24]

This is the nub of all rights talk, all talk of abomination, liberation, or resistance. Without the real existence of human persons as moral agents, without an understanding of what constitutes human persons, without seeing that human persons must have *capacities* for communication, interpretation, rational discourse, or self-creation, none of these privileged topics can have any meaning.

Bernstein, like some other contemporary philosophers, tries to establish bridges of continuity between quite divergent philosophical positions in the United States and Europe. There is some question, however, whether many academic philosophers will admit that the only bridge possible is a humanly built one.

In contemporary philosophical debate, one can find the same pattern of approach and avoidance that characterizes our personal and social lives. Some cannot find the person; some wish not to; some forbid even the looking. And some persist.

Let us join those who so persist. Let us remember, however, that all philosophical discourse—ethics all the more so—must be true to the human subject from which it springs. Both must be true to the only experience that gave them birth: the experience of real men and women questioning themselves and their world.

THE TEXTURE OF PERSONAL REALITY
AND ETHICAL EXPERIENCE

American phenomenologist Calvin Schrag, in *Experience and Being*, has argued that all philosophical enterprises must be grounded in experience as a complex, multi-dimensional dynamic field, to which all inquiry must return and refer. One can have no starting place other than the world-attached, experiencing person who questions. Moreover, to start is to be inserted into the dynamic field itself, made up of inseparable constituents: the experiencer (subject)-experiencing-a figure (object)-in a ground (context).[25]

By calling human experience a "field," we attend to the fact that the totality cannot be understood without relation to all of the parts and that no one of the parts can be understood without its relation to the other parts, all dynamically related and influencing each other. A baseball field, for example, is hopelessly incomprehensible if you try to understand it by focusing on one "part" as the entire mystery of the whole game. Pitching by itself does not unpack the mystery of baseball. In fact, pitching—or batting, for that matter—has no intelligibility without fielders, batters, innings, outs, and countless other components that are intimately interrelated. You must understand the whole thing to understand the parts. Yet the only way to get to the whole thing is through the parts. We always start and end, however, with the whole dynamic reality. That whole is what Hegel and Marx called a "dialectical" totality.

Schrag's insight cannot be stressed enough—especially for people undertaking an investigation into ethics. We enter the very realm of moral life and philosophy as inescapably human, *as* multi-dimensional persons who (a) have the subjective endowments required to dynamically experience our interior world, (b) are always set in a background of personal history and context, and (c) inhabit life under the objective conditions of this cosmos and an intersubjective world of language and tradition. Therefore, our subsequent investigation must (a) look into the very conditions for the possibility of being personal selves, (b) attend to our historical and cultural embeddedness, and (c) honor the objective conditions of our bodies in a world independent of our intentions.

It is always possible—and often desirable—to concentrate on one or another component of our experience and submit it to secondary analysis. The integrated totality of personal experience must always be the starting and ending point, however.

No aspect or component of our experience should be shut off from investigation a priori. Every aspect of our conscious engagement of life is worth attending to. Everything counts. We must refuse to close off data.

The human who philosophizes, who does ethics, cannot escape the body and the skin of his or her humanity, cannot leap out of context, cannot pretend to be "non"-self-conscious, cannot take the posture of being ahistorical, and cannot repress the objective dimensions of experience.

Nothing of experience should be repressed. No question should be stifled—especially the foundational questions that make ethics possible in the first place. Any philosophy that would make us repress the questions of our identity and our action must be considered a negation not only of ethics but of our very humanity.

A human ethics must be open to consideration of anything that is human: open to experience, open to the demands that human questioning makes of us, and open to an understanding of what makes questioning possible in the first place. That experiential openness is not only what makes ethics possible; it is what makes mature human experience possible.

The ethical question, like the human asking it, is an historical reality, situated in space and time—a practical moment of choice. It is unavoidably incarnate, enfleshed, and local. Thus, anyone who has rejected antiquated schemes of "autonomous man" or the "ahistorical subject" or the "isolated imperial self" is right to do so. Variations of the Cartesian-Humean ego were invariably either monadic or nomadic:

There was either nothing outside our minds or nothing in them. There was either no world to go out to or no place to come home to. The great masters of suspicion—whether the troubled old-timers Freud or Nietzsche (who will always have something to say to the human mind and to move the human heart) or the fashionably obstreperous Derrida and Foucault—may be the necessary purgatory for vaunted modern pride. They have played their role in our disillusionment, in our acquisition of a more humble and chastened understanding of ourselves: creatures, whether we like it or not, of history and culture.

Not only that, however: What liberates us from being mere hapless creatures of culture and passive victims of history is that we can mount a self-critical questioning of our particular space and time. We can own or disown our history. Some of us actually become Humes, Derridas, Freuds, and Carol Gilligans who introduce a different voice to tired discourse.

Knowing ourselves as contextualized, we can accept and own ourselves as persons, selves, humans—no matter what our context. Herein we are able to speak across cultures, criticize them, and arbitrate them. We appropriate our time and history as *ours*.

Thus, as persons, as ethical beings, as questioners, we throw the immediate world into question. Although our question is always limited in and through time, it is nonetheless a liberating act of disengagement from fixed history. The very meaning of the ethical question is to challenge the fixity of the given here and now and to ask what is *not*. Ethical questions distance and free us from unquestioning passive acceptance. They liberate us from a forcibly imposed world.

When we first ask ourselves the question of moral action, we experience the birth of responsibility. We are experiencing the emergence of ethics. We are getting in touch with what it means to be a person, to live life as a person. Moreover, every ethical question we pose—as well as the strategic world that flows from it—has the time-bound flesh and blood of the person who poses it. We are not dealing with some "ahistorical" self here. We *are* selves, indeed—but we are flesh, incarnate in space and time.

Yet the very fact that we do question ourselves here and now frees us in space and time. The moment we ask a moral question, we disengage from blind acceptance of the way things are here and now. We are flesh, but we are conscious of the fact. We even take ownership of it.

A truly human ethics, like the human persons who introduce it to the world, is a multi-dimensional inquiry. It is a human enterprise, preeminently personal, embodied in space and time, self-consciously incarnate.

A multi-dimensional life of embodied self-consciousness is what ethics is all about because that is what persons are all about. Persons are not isolated individuals or theoretical constructs but living, historical creatures, in touch with their humanity in its brokenness and aspiration. These are the beings whose disappearance Walker Percy mourns. Theirs is the density and richness of personal life that seems so absent from the media-constructed life of a Donald Trump. These are the flesh and blood persons whom Derek Parfit apparently thinks "do not matter."

3
Personal Bodies

I distinguished two views about the nature of a person. On the
nonreductionist view, a person is a separately existing entity, distinct
from his brain and body and his experiences. On the best-known
version of this view, a person is a Cartesian Ego. . . .

What I find is this. I can believe [the reductionist view] at the
intellectual or reflective level. I am convinced by the arguments in favor
of this view. But I think it likely that, at some other level, I shall always
have doubts. My belief is firmest when I am considering some of these
imagined cases.

Derek Parfit[1]

Will identity survive? Can it *develop* in face of such a shattering, such
pressures—or will it be overwhelmed, to produce a "Tourettized soul"
(in the poignant words of a patient I was later to see)? There is a
physiological, and existential, almost a theological pressure upon the
soul of the Touretter—whether it can be held whole and sovereign, or
whether it will be taken over, possessed and dispossessed, by every
immediacy and impulse. Hume, as we have noted, wrote: "I venture to
affirm . . . that we are nothing but a bundle or collection of different
sensations, succeeding one another with inconceivable rapidity, and in a
perpetual flux and movement." Thus, for Hume, personal identity is a
fiction—we do not exist, we are but a consecution of sensations, or
perceptions. This is clearly not the case with a normal human being,
because he *owns* his own perceptions. They are not a mere flux, but *his*
own, united by an abiding individuality or self. But what Hume describes
may be precisely the case for a being as unstable as a super-Touretter,
whose life is, to some extent, a consecution of random or convulsive
perceptions and motions, a phantasmagoric fluttering with no center or
sense. To this extent he *is* a "Humean" rather than a human being.

Oliver Sacks[2]

The Unity of man has not yet been broken; the body has not been stripped of human predicates; it has not yet become a machine; and the soul has not yet been defined as existence for-itself (*pour soi*). Naïve consciousness does not see in the soul the *cause* of the movement of the body nor does it put the soul in the body as the pilot in his ship. This way of thinking belongs to philosophy; it is not implied in immediate experience.
Maurice Merleau-Ponty[3]

ON THE MATTER AND SPIRIT OF MAPS

If ethical behavior and ethical studies emerge only from the questioning of persons, we must examine the reality of human personhood. The investigation must not be limited, however, by any prior "mapping" of human reality that will exclude possible findings. Starting with some partial or constricted map for our experience that would eliminate at the outset any aspect of personal existence would be foolish.

For example, upon his father's return from a journey to India, a young boy brings a globe to the kitchen table. He wants his dad to point out on the map where he had been. The globe is turned to the Asian sub-continent, where India is marked. "But where in India?" the boy inquires. Then the dots of Madras, Calcutta, and Bangalore are pointed out.

"So, where are we?"

With a turn of the earth, the United States comes into view; after further questions that bring us to the dot of St. Louis, the boy asks, "Where is the kitchen?"

"It's not on the map."

The boy's face falls in disappointment. It's almost as if his most real and familiar experience has no confirmation in the world. He is finally consoled when his father draws a map of their house, indicates the kitchen table, and then tells the boy that India cannot be found on this map either—but that doesn't make India nonexistent.

We cannot possibly find what our maps for investigation do not include. This notion should warn us that in our investigations into the matters of human questioning and action, we must be wary of maps that exclude our very humanness.

Derek Parfit's impressive work *Reasons and Persons* has attracted considerable scholarly attention. Nonetheless it is a seriously limited map. It represents many of the more frustrating impulses in contemporary philosophy. The frustration is not directed at the elegance and pursuit of the argument; the problem is the map Parfit presents.

Parfit provides us with only two views of the human person. The first is what he calls a "nonreductionist view," all variations of which are apparently squeezed into a Cartesian Ego—a "person" somehow distinct from brain, body, and experience. This map collapses the rich multi-dimensionality of personal reality into a cognitive and disembodied being. What might such a thing be? Where on earth might it be found? The only other acceptable map available in Parfit's account of personal reality is that "our existence just involves the existence of our brains and bodies, and the doing of our deeds, and the thinking of our thoughts, and the occurrence of certain other physical and mental events."[4] For Parfit, this grid is reductionist and materialist. Because the implications of the dualist option are supposedly preposterous, we are presented with no other choice than Parfit's materialism over Descartes' disembodied phantom.

This offering of only two maps is a spurious dichotomy, a false dilemma. It is like being presented with two and only two schemas of the world, one providing altitudes and the other population density, and being told that there is no rainfall on the earth.

The big journey through Parfit's book is commendable. In this work as well as the work of others who do "philosophy of mind," however, the maps we usually are permitted to use are too constricting. It is almost impossible to find any coordinates to locate notions of substance and nature or our experience of being animals, reflexively conscious of ourselves. There is no habitat provided for phenomenology or the experience of the lived body. There are no alternative routes offered for the human journey other than those of Descartes and Hume.[5] More problematic yet, there is little that makes sense to an ordinarily intelligent person.

Parfit does seem to acknowledge a discomfort with this forced option. "At some other level," he says, there are nagging doubts. That "other" level may well be life itself; the doubts may be those that stalk any philosopher who starts with a map that closes off too many explorations at the outset. A theoretician with a pinched map of existence can be as uncomfortable as a child who cannot find the kitchen on a map of nations.[6]

Parfit tells us (in the lead quotation of this chapter) that his doubts are eased when he entertains "imagined cases" of androids, body-machines, teletransportation, and weird self-divisions. This attitude might strike most humans as a strange and strained consolation. Admittedly, such thought experiments and imagined fantasies can be serviceable, possibly in the testing out of claims that are made. It is puzzling, however, that one rarely finds an equal amount of devotion to the lived experience of a mature human that one finds in discussions about clever machines, brain transplants, and out-of-body experiences.[7]

Attempting to explain our embodied consciousness only in terms of a Cartesian ego is like searching for the kitchen table on a map of continents: It will end up nowhere. The same fate awaits anyone who proposes to explain personal experience exclusively in terms of non-conscious quantifiable operations: They will be as successful as people looking for Africa on a map of the kitchen.

A multiplicity of maps is desirable, of course. Diverse maps allow us to concentrate on secondary topics of experience and give specialized understanding to the various parts of our make-up as human beings. The only map that will be finally adequate in helping us comprehend what we are, however, is one capacious enough not to repress or ignore any part of our personal existence.

ON THE MATTER AND SPIRIT OF PERSONS

The neurologist Oliver Sacks deals with persons. He refuses to impose any preordained grid of theory on the living patient. Thus, when he reflects about seriously neurologically damaged persons—in the case of the second featured quotation at the beginning of this chapter, a man suffering from the chaos of Tourette's syndrome, with its symptomatic clatter of impulsive, unconnected spasms of language and affect—Sacks finds it odd that David Hume's philosophical rendition of selfhood best fits the maelstrom of a Touretter's soul rather than an ordinary, more fully functioning person.

Hume wrote, "I venture to affirm . . . that [we] are nothing but a bundle or collection of different sensations, succeeding one another with inconceivable rapidity, and in a perpetual flux and movement."[8] For Sacks, however, the very quality that characterizes human identity— a capacity for integrated ownership of words, experiences, and affections—is absent from Hume's famous passage—and from his understanding of the human person. The most damaged human is most like a "*Humean*" being—precisely because of the damage.

Even the Touretter, however, fights to maintain some personally integrated individuality under the onslaught of fragmentation. Sacks tells us that despite the most daunting barriers to individuation and realized personhood, the Touretter succeeds in most cases. "For the powers of survival, of the will to survive, and to survive as a unique inalienable individual, are, absolutely, the strongest in our being; stronger than any impulses, stronger than disease."[9]

Our power to survive as unique inalienable individuals is one with what and who we are. We are embodied, self-consciously endowed animals, subject to space and history; as the next chapter demonstrates, such endowments make us personal animals and moral agents.

The map of Oliver Sacks—even as a neurologist—ranges over the primary terrain of human inquiry: It is the human person engaging a human world. Sacks, of course, values and contributes to the secondary mapping of human behavior in physical, chemical, and anatomical models. He begins and ends, however, at the ground of human experience—the only place any human being can enter the world.

This is the way that we are given to ourselves: not as ghosts in machines, not as machines without a ghost, but as embodied, self-conscious unities.

Here emerges the option that Merleau-Ponty offers in the third quote at the beginning of this chapter. In effect, Merleau-Ponty reminds us of our beginnings. He gives us a map of reality that does not exclude the insights of a Hume or a Descartes or the challenges of a Derek Parfit—but also does not repress the flesh-and-blood self-conscious reality of these men. Nor does it restrict the questions we are allowed to ask or confine us only to privileged roads of investigation.

Our immediate experience of ourselves in the world is a unity prior to brokenness, prior to a delusion that we must be either of two isolated substances, soul and body, that somehow must now, by philosophical conjuring, be brought together. Thus, a human body is not some outside "thing," some instrument, or some machine inhabited by a ghost: "It is our expression in the world, the visible form of our intentions."[10]

The work of Merleau-Ponty and other phenomenologists suggests the most appropriate mapping for our ethical search. Although his way is not the only way, it is a more inclusive way—broad enough and inclusive enough that nothing of human import is closed off or omitted *a priori* in our investigation. The work of any scientist, logician, artist, or linguist is a value to such a map. The undertaking of philosophy cannot be jammed into the limited categories or questions that only a particular kind of scientist, logician, artist, or linguist might employ, however. We must begin with the living, engaged-in-the-world person.

PERSONAL EMBODIMENT

We are in the world as self-conscious bodies. We find ourselves in the middle of lives that are urgent to us, lives that are morally and existentially significant. That is the only way we know any world at all.

Choosing embodiment as a starting point is not a claim of isolation or atomic separateness from the world or others. The words we use, the texts we write, even the way we *approach* words and texts is set in coordinates of space and time, mediated to us by culture and intersubjective discourse. Similarly, investigations into neuroanatomy and brain deficits reveal crucial *components* of our experience. They all emerge from and impinge on us, however, as embodied and self-conscious living beings.

The emphasis on the body is most important, especially if one is tempted to identify the human person with mental states or the brain itself. The luminous work of neurologist Antonio Damasio exhibits this concern for embodiment, although it does not share the natural endowment theory I propose. In *The Feeling of What Happens: Body and Emotion in the Making of Consciousness*, Damasio seeks to correct the "noticeable absence of a notion of *organism* in cognitive science and neuroscience. The mind remained linked to the brain in a somewhat equivocal relationship, and the brain remained consistently separated from the body rather than being seen as part of a complex living organism."[11] Thus, his investigation into human consciousness is marked by rich case studies, allusions to poetry and music, and patients' phenomenological descriptions of their trauma and loss.

For my own purposes, I offer a phenomenological description that is open to confirmation or rejection by any reader. My description is congruent in many ways with Damasio's neurology, though I am more influenced by the approach and style of Merleau-Ponty (a philosopher whom Damasio himself mentions as providing a precedent for the idea that the body is a basis for the self).[12]

I cannot begin speaking, writing, acting, or thinking without beginning self-consciously and bodily. The task of ethics, as well as all questions about personal agency, whether approached through language, tradition, obligation, or nature, cannot get underway if there is no historically situated, self-conscious questioner to launch it.

The ethical question is put to me only because I have the ability to focus on my own consciousness and therefore become morally problematic to myself. I could not even begin an ethical investigation if I were not a subject of experience—an "I" arranged and deployed for action over space and time. Nor could I be concerned with what I might do or what course of action I might take if I did not in some way have ownership of my consciousness and my body as my own.

My ethical questions partake of the quality of my own existence, from which they spring. Any moral choice I make and the question it pulls from me are inescapably historical: like me, lodged in space and time, contextualized by countless relationships and structures.

There would be no ethical act, no study of ethics, if there were no moment of time in which choice might occur, or no history, or no narrative of my own self-interpretation. There would be no ethics if there were no reflectively conscious beings to make self-narration possible.[13]

My being human, my embodied-self-consciousness, is the arena of and condition for ethics. Therefore to understand ethics, I must first understand the personal ground from which it grows, the soil of my own space—history aware of itself, the soil of embodiment.

This is not Kant's "transcendental unity of apperception"; it is not Descartes' "I think"; it is not Hume's observer or receiver. I am and have *embodied* reflexive consciousness.

We are immediately and unassailably given to ourselves and the world as structured in space and time and as being self-consciously aware of it. This recognition is not the result of a demonstration or deduction. I cannot "find," "come to," "discover," or observe the very condition that makes observation and discovery possible. The evidence is its givenness—vulnerable before doubt only because everything human is open to doubt.

BODY AS OBJECT, BODY AS SUBJECT

When I experience my body as my own, as me, I do not experience it as an object. Indeed, there are times that I may approach or approximate experiencing the sheer structure or materiality of my body as an object—but that is only in moments of disintegration, conscious distancing and discipline, physical sickness, or alienation.

In nausea or anesthesia, I may experience the body more in its "objectiveness" and "otherness." This is the "it-ness" of my body—without which, as Martin Buber has said, we cannot live. As I faint, as I "lose" consciousness, I experience the object-ness of the body, its falling into thing-ness, even catching the echo of lost embodied subjectivity.

I may even self-consciously put my body at a cognitive distance— as I study anatomy, practice yoga postures, or engage biofeedback to quiet pain. I can also partially objectify my body—still experienced as mine—through intention as I practice physical discipline and training. Thus, my fingers resist the endless arpeggios of guitar finger-picking or piano paces. My physicalness fights the intentions of diving gainers, ice-skating Salchows, or the trapping of a soccer ball in my waist.

In some ways, I can even find my body "distanced" or somehow separated from my ownness as another person stares, looks me over, prods me. I can even fall into the illusion—whether induced by my own psychohistory or programmed by cultural propaganda—that my body is some thing: a commodity, an albatross, a curse. Those moments of dis-ease and dis-integration actually illuminate my normal and opaque existence. They are dramatic *contrasts* to our everyday lived experience of being fully embodied.

I presume, expect, and rely on the daily unquestioned experience of embodied self-conscious unity. I could not even go on talking, writing, hoping, feeling, and loving without such a presupposition. The *dis*-unity surprises and disorients me; the *breakdown* of the unity incapacitates me.

To be a human person is to experience the fragility of an integrated, self-conscious, embodied unity. It also is to experience the thrall of powerful unities.

There are the stunning moments of reintegration: the effortless flight, the thrilling execution of movement, the ecstasy of interpenetrating physicality and spirit. Full embodiment is union. Thus, we become our very hands when the arpeggios are mastered. One's leaping body becomes one's self. One's expression in art is one's being actualized. A physical breakthrough becomes a personal release: Resistance is no longer felt in the pure self-expression of a masterful swan dive, the ice-dancing of Torvill and Dean, the embodied grace of gymnastics. The body in these unifications feels, seems, almost *is* intelligence. The body embodies, expresses, reveals self-consciousness. Word is fully fleshed, and my flesh is personal utterance.

Thus, all of the aforementioned experiences of "objectness" are contrasts, not only to the highest experiences of embodiment but also to the everyday givenness of it: in the touch, in the spring of a step, in the encountering of another face, in the sigh. These experiences are not alienating, as it might be when we are reduced to the sheer physicality of the body. They do, however, reveal how we are, in some ways, physical objects.

Yet the human body, though structured and objectifiable in embodiment, is not an object. It is physical subjectivity—mine, me, myself. An embodied experience is an experience of our bodies, willy nilly, as *ours*, as *ourselves*, as our subjectivity in time whereby we are invited into the world and we are able to enter the world. Our bodies are our invitations to life. They also are Life's invitation to us. We enter life; life enters us, as self-conscious, embodied beings. Embodiment is not the experience of one's body as an "it." It is the experience of one's body as oneself. My body is me. Your body is you.

My body always reveals more than itself as an object. As sheer body-object, it would be corpse. As embodiment, however, it reveals me as a subject of life. It is my primary and first expression to the world. My body is a revealing, an utterance. I experience it as my word-in-flesh, intrinsic to my own life-narrative. My body is my self-conscious revelation, expressing me, unveiling me in space and time. My body is the very personalization of this reality I know as me—the condition for my possibility as a person in the world of nature, things, and memory.

We can examine personal embodiment—what it seems to be made of, how it is experienced as a unity, and what conditions and endowments make it possible. This examination would be in many ways a hermeneutics of the body, available only to a self-interpreting and expressing being. This we will do.

First, however, let us acknowledge the body's ambivalences. The human person is not two things glued together, a hodge-podge of independent pluralities, or a hybrid of two beings. Yet there are ambivalences in what we are. Embodiment—human personhood—before any analysis is freighted with paradox, even ambiguity.

AMBIGUITIES OF EMBODIMENT

Opened and Closed

As bodied, I experience myself as being open to the world. I am made available to space and history. The only way to find me is to locate me in time, to spot my body, in the here and now. As bodied, then, I am actual. I am some body. Somebody. Because I am bodied, the world of space-time is available for me.

Yet because of the very fact of my body, I experience myself as apart from the world, even though I am part of it. Although my body is my availability to the world, as bodied, my availability is held in check.

I do not intend this ambiguity as a confirmation of a position often attributed to Plato—that our bodies are prisons or cages, from which we will be released (although this side of the ambiguity could provide some evidence to lead to such a conclusion). No: The ambiguous phenomenon of the body is precisely the occasion of historical limitation and liberation at the same time. As embodied, I am unleashed, freed to history; as embodied, I am confined to it.

Even this ambiguity is not the final word because the ambiguity is resolved in fuller circles of embodied action wherein the conditions of body-limits become the very expressions of transcending those limits.

A Part and Apart

In embodiment I experience my body as the way of unity and communion. I am one with the world, inextricably a part of it. I am available for unity with you, with others, with any part of the world in the mediations of bodily presence. We speak, we touch, we offer grasps of assistance, grips of solidarity. One makes love in body action, and one makes the culture in labor with another. We make words into flesh and flesh into words. We give intent, passion, spirit to material reality.

Yet in embodiment I am immediately in a position of separateness and apartness. Apart, as my body, I can never be wholly a part of you. Even our most vaunted and valued attempts at union carry the bitter-sweetness of exhausting attempts at overcoming separateness, of fully communicating, of utter communion. We fall back, daunted by the limitedness of expression. Precisely as embodied, as body, we collide with impenetrable barriers.

I am prevented from being fully with and in you, in your space and time, by the very phenomenon of embodiment that offers union in the first place.

Uncovered and Hidden

Embodiment is revelation. It shows me forth. It shows me up. It may even show me off. Embodying in gesture, word, movement, arch of eye, and tone of voice, I reveal that mystery of consciousness in space and time that is my personhood. Embodiment is expression, interpretation, communication, and language—all at once and primarily.

Yet embodiment is concealment. Not only is my body inadequate as a manifestation of all I am: It hides all I am. Even though I am transparent and accessible to you (as well as myself) as embodied, I am at the same time opaque and covert. My uncovering, my very embodiment is my cover. My self-revelations also hide me.

The ugliness of Jean Paul Sartre shared the painful ambivalence of Marilyn Monroe's ravishing beauty. Both experienced their respective appearances as a paradox of revelation and concealment.

Free and Limited

As embodiment, I am actual. As body, I am here. I am now—to be some body.

As embodied I am merely and only here, however—merely now and only once. As embodied, I am. I am in limit. My body is my existence and my nonexistence at the same time.

By the body I freely engage history. I achieve historicity. I elaborate the drama of my life—a self-narrating narrative. I am some how, somewhere. As embodied I am unleashed into space and time. Yet the very condition of my historical actuality is the determinateness of situation. To be free to history is to be somehow stuck in it. The living human body is an openness in space and time and a confinement in space and time.

This is the paradox of embodiment's limited engagement. I am in a place! But only here. I am in time! But only now. I am actual! Somebody! But merely some *body*. Only *some*. As embodied I find myself only in *this* place and time. Self-consciously aware of it, however, time and space are *mine*—to act in, to live through.

The privilege of embodiment is to *be* something. Its price is not to be *everything*—to be limited. Through those limits, however, one might be open to all that has no limits but is expressed, revealed, and communicated through them.

Openness and closedness, unity and separateness, revelation and concealment, freedom and determinateness are the ambiguities, then, of finding ourselves as embodied self-consciousnesses. They are the paradoxes of embodiment; as such, they are the marks of every other human self-revelation: language, culture, labor, and gesture. These are the ambiguities that, Calvin Schrag has cautioned, can tempt us with false dichotomics. They lead to alienation and the loss of embodied integrity if we insist on being *either* pure consciousness for itself *or* sheer animal in itself. These paradoxes, as we shall see, also are the conditions of our knowledge and freedom.

THE "MY-NESS" AND "ME-NESS" OF A PERSONAL BODY

There is a certain artificiality in speaking of "embodiment" without some constant acknowledgment and even development of the subjective "my-ness" of the experience. None of the discussion about "my" body could even be uttered, much less conceived, if my body were not experienced as "mine," if there were not something about me whereby I experience my body as self-revealing.

Antonio Damasio offers a lucid and elegant account of this experience:

> The sensory images of what you perceive externally, and the related images you recall, occupy most of the scope of your mind, but not all of it. Besides those images there is also this other presence that signifies you, as observer of the things imaged, owner of the things imaged, potential actor on the things imaged. There is a presence of you in a particular relationship with some object. If there were no such presence, how would your thoughts belong to you? Who could tell that they did? The presence is quiet and subtle, and sometimes it is little more than a "hint half guessed," a "gift half understood," to borrow words from T.S. Eliot.[14]

Whereas Damasio proposes a neurological rendition of this "feeling of what happens," I propose that the key to embodied experiences as "mine" is reflexive consciousness—an activity we will fully examine later on but we can initially understand as an *awareness of being aware* of oneself as body. My experiencing of myself as a person in the world has an inescapable complexity, to be sure, but there is also an inescapably unified givenness of it as being "mine."

I do not mean this in the sense of property-ownership or in the sense that this reflexive awareness is the real "I" that is somehow directing or ordering my body around. I mean it in the sense that I am aware of being a center of bodied experience—made available by reflexive awareness—and thereby capable of taking an attitude toward myself and the world, questioning both and being in some ways accountable in relationship to both.

Although there is ambiguity in the experience of embodiment, there are not "two worlds" about it. There is just one world I experience—the world of a personal body: the lived, experiencial alternative to the forced option that we have encountered in Parfit's *Reasons and Persons*. We experience ourselves as unified realities—not split but integrated, multi-dimensional beings.

A hallmark of the inheritors of Hume has been that their map of human existence has no room for such a notion of embodiment. Gilbert Ryle, for example, in his famous *The Concept of Mind*, prepared us for the contemporary quandary that Parfit represents when he located the nonreductionist position in the official doctrine of "the Cartesian Myth." Here, literally, is a never-never land wherein "a person therefore lives through two collateral histories, one consisting of what happens in and to his body, the other consisting of what happens in and to his mind."[15]

This is a false gambit—attempted before and after Ryle—that serves only to bypass consideration of the human person as embodied and self-reflexive. No alternative is offered us other than disembodied minds and demented bodies. Ryle rejects—and rightly so—a rigid dualism of independent entities somehow stuck together but never experienced as human.[16] If one is forced to accept the choice between pure mind and utter body, however, the human person is lost.

There are many definitions of the self in current use: It is relational, it is linguistic, it is social, it is historical, it is developmental. All, in a sense, are true. Unless you have a *being*, however, capacitated for society, language, and mutuality, there can be no derived notions of a human self. In the deepest sense of the word, the "self" to which I refer when I say "myself" is the embodied career.

Even the great Kierkegaard—possibly as far from Ryle as one might be—in his famous beginning of *Sickness Unto Death* seems to fall into the forced option of a hermetic self:

> Man is spirit. But what is spirit? Spirit is the self. But what is the self? The self is a relation which relates itself to its own self, or it is that in the relation (which accounts for it) that the relation relates itself to its own self; the self is not the relation but (consists in the fact) that the relation relates itself to his ownself.[17]

True, Kierkegaard forces us to confront the issue of reflexivity and its relation to selfhood, but his framing of the issue suggests a Cartesian split of the human person—that the self is actually spirit, rather than incarnate spirit. Thus, it oddly supports Ryle's portrayal of the mind-body double-world thesis. The lived personal body—with all its ambiguity, actuality, temporality, and spatiality—does not appear here.

Yet the embodied, self-conscious world is the only one we inhabit. Human beings, human selves, human persons are not "spirits" or souls, although they may *have* both. They may not indeed be "ahistorical" selves, but they are personal beings—embodied, self-conscious human careers—that can take ownership of and transcend their history.

To repeat, the act and endowment of pure reflexivity is not the "self" but a capacity of personal animals, empowering them to relate to their history and space *as* selves. To miss this point is to entertain the illusion that the "self" or "autonomous man" or "transcendent Ego" (or, more contemporaneously, "brain" or "mind") is somehow magically separated from the actual living human organism and somehow got attached through the pineal gland (or arrived at that magical moment when we started having conscious states). This conceptual prison confines much talk about the "mind-body" problem.

The search for a disembodied human self has lurched to a dead end. The "autonomous" ego with no history, no communal ties, and no "place" has not been sighted. It is this "man" whose end has been announced, whose "self" has been unmasked, whose ego has become decentered.

The embodied, self-conscious person has not. "The man Kierkegaard," Unamuno would say, and "the flesh-and-blood Gilbert Ryle" are both embodied, self-conscious persons inhabiting only one world. It is that world, with them, that each of us must start with.

Kierkegaard, however, does investigate—and masterfully so—what many others ignore: the fact of reflexive consciousness.[18] This fact renders our bodies and all our embodied expressions personal. The consciousness that I have of writing now is a consciousness of this activity as mine. The embodiment or expression of writing is related to me as a center of consciousness revealed in and through this, its act. Thus, it is with any experience of community, any encounter with "otherness," any interpretation that I may make of myself or the world, and any questioning I may address to reality. Certainly my experience of embodied subjectivity is mediated by culture, language, genetics—but I encounter none of them if I am not a living human person doing so.[19]

My body and all my embodiments are revelations of me. They are my responsive expressions to the world and my place in it; as self-consciously responsive, I am the originator of them. They reveal my agency in ways that are not automatic, forced, or necessitated but (as we shall see) limited in freedom. Personal agency, then, is not just behavior or activity. Nor is it merely a revelation of the *kind* of being I am, as dog behavior reveals dogness or a machine "reveals" what it is and does. Human action also reveals the individual person's self-definition and self-revelation. It reveals a human project freely given.

My actions reveal not only my humanity; they reveal the kind of human I am as well. They reveal how I, with some degree of self-possession, stand in relationship to the world. They are, one might say, my "self-utterance." As Gerard Manley Hopkins wrote:

Each mortal thing does one thing and the same:
Deals out that being indoors each one dwells;
Selves—goes itself; *myself* it speaks and spells,
Crying *What I do is me: for that I came.*
I say more: the just man justices . . .[20]

All personal actions are embodiments, self-revelations. They are the primordial expressions of persons. Ethics, in this basic sense, is embodiment. Ethics is self-expression. It is self-interpreting revelation.

PERSONAL CONSCIOUSNESS

What is Kierkegaard getting at when he describes a relation that relates itself to its own self? It is reflexive consciousness—a knowledge that knows itself, relates to itself, in the act of knowing. Thomas Aquinas appealed to this kind of consciousness when he described the remarkable capacities for intimacy and depth that humans exhibit.[21] This consciousness is the condition for the possibility of all discussions about the self. It also is the phenomenon theoreticians most commonly ignore when they propose to explain human behavior entirely in physical terms.[22]

There is world. There are bodies. There also is awareness of the world, awareness of bodies. If that were all, there would still be no human selves, no humanly developing persons. In the experience of myself as embodied, however, there is an act of awareness that is not simply awareness of the world or objects or body sensations of the world. There is additionally—and crucially—an act of awareness that turns back upon itself and is aware of itself in being aware of the world.

This act of reflexive awareness is not the "I," nor is it the phenomenon of embodiment; yet it makes both possible. It is not my "reflecting" about my life, conduct, or self but the reflexive act of personal consciousness that makes all of those possible.

This act of reflexive awareness, which is available to any self, may be called "awareness of awareness," "consciousness of consciousness," "reflexive consciousness," or "concomitant consciousness." I abbreviate it as A2 (standing for "awareness of awareness" and its equivalents).

A2 is neither the self nor the person, but it is *of* the personal animal. It is an endowment of human beings capacitated to be personal selves, whereby the experience of selfhood is made possible. A2 is not required for a living body to be responsive and reactive to the world and other bodies. Surely animals (and possibly plants and other organisms, as Damasio suggests) interact with the world this way. A2, however, is a required constitutive dimension of embodiment, whereby a body is experienced as one's own subjectivity in the world.[23]

Thus, I find myself, among the bodies of the world, as one endowed with a capacity to be aware of my own awareness of the world and to enter into relationship to this awareness as my own. This capacitates me to interpret my experienced world, to question it, and to communicate with it.

I do not know how awareness could be wholly and only aware of its own act of awareness, without any other content but its own awareness. I, as human, *always* require content in my acts of reflexive consciousness. All of my knowing is inescapably embodied because all of my cognitive endowments, with all other manifold capacities, are of and by a body-person.

Although A2 is not the same as one's self or person, it makes possible the *emergence* of psychological and social "selfhood" over time. As such, it is the source of subjectivity, the experience of being a "subject." It is not some hidden and autonomous subject behind the body, however. The whole body-person is the subject. Without body, a human person would be some other kind of being than a human being; without A2, the human body could not be the occasion of "embodiment." It would be like all other animals.

Finally, being reflexively aware is not the same as being an "overly sensitive," highly "self-conscious" person concerned with the way one "comes across" to others. It is not an intentional and intensive focus that must be "turned on" or brought to our behaviors. Although we need not—and ought not—always attend to A2, it is always present in our knowing, whether we are awake or dreaming. It also may be constantly present to our very being because this conscious reflexivity makes possible the experience of being and having "my body."

PERSONALIZED WORLD

"Awareness" of the world in a nonpersonal fashion may be possible. Indeed, perhaps every object or individual being has a primitive form of awareness in the sense of being reactive and capable of entering into bonds—in subatomic particles, molecules, or organisms.

Even more, animals surely have an awareness that they experience as sensation—the reception of particular and concrete cues, the integration and storage of them, the retrieval of them. We ourselves might imagine having such pure sensations, without any reflexive consciousness of them. Aristotle's discussion of the internal and external sensations is remarkably prescient in this regard. His attribution of sense memory, sense imagination, and sense-unified awareness to the cortex of the brain has been confirmed by the best neural technology and research of our time.[24]

There is another awareness of the world, however, whereby it becomes "mine." Not that I possess the world in any propertied sense but that it becomes *for me* just as I become a reality *for myself*. I enter into relation to the world, question it, interpret it. I do this because I am capable of a consciousness that relates to itself in being conscious of the world.

Neurosurgeon Wilder Penfield witnessed such a phenomenon dramatically in his early experiments probing the human cortex by electrodes.

> Consider the point of view of the patient when the surgeon's electrode, placed on the interpretive cortex, summons the replay of past experience. The stream of consciousness is suddenly doubled for him. He is aware of what is going on in the operating room as well as the "flashback" from the past. He can discuss with the surgeon the meaning of both streams.
>
> The patient's mind, which is considering the situation in such an aloof and critical manner, can only be something quite apart from neuronal reflex action. It is noteworthy that two streams of consciousness are flowing, one driven by input from environment, the other by an electrode delivering sixty pulses per second to the cortex. The fact that there should be no confusion in the conscious state suggests that, although the content of consciousness depends in large measure on neuronal activity, awareness itself does not.[25]

What Penfield describes as "awareness" (what I have been calling A2) is a part of the patient's experience that is not reducible to the two different "contents" or streams of consciousness that are intrinsically modified by the probing of the brain.

Indeed the "person," the "self," who is the "patient" is profoundly affected by the structure, input, and processes of the brain triggered by the immediately sensed environment as well as the probing of the electrodes. The awareness of awareness, in relation to the various inputs, considered in itself, is not.

Our endowment of reflexive consciousness persists through the most serious of brain deficits and assaults on the brain—even if there is minimal or unobserved neuronal activity and supply of content.

The reflexive capacity of A2 enables the human person to self-consciously relate to his or her world even in the midst of profound damage to the person's body and brain. Thus, Oliver Sacks' *Clinical Tales* are startling accounts of people who haltingly affirm the "I," whether they are beset with massive memory loss, have autism affect deficiencies, or are even unable to remember what happened to them five minutes previously.

The PBS series *The Mind* related a particularly poignant example (later recounted in Richard Restak's volume of the same title). A brilliant composer had lost all capacity to remember any information for more than five minutes. He clearly has a self, a conscious presence to his own consciousness; yet a debilitating encephalitis has damaged his cortex so profoundly that there is no thematic content to his memory for him to be aware of. He spends his days playing solitaire and making endless entries into a notebook. The entries read: "Now I am completely aware, for the first time in years." His wife attempts to describe how he seems to experience his own selfhood: "Clive's world now consists of a moment, with no past to anchor it and no future to look ahead. It's a blinkered moment." Yet Clive's struggle for a unified sense of self, even without the content of the past, is as striking as the cases recounted by Oliver Sacks. His wife continues: "His being, his center, his soul is absolutely functioning as it ever did. The fact that he is so despairing, so much in anguish, so angry, so much in love with me—those are real, human passions. And he is showing them almost to the exclusion of everything else."[26]

Despite massive compromises to our brains—comas, deficits of external sensation, "split personalities," even hemispherectomy—there remains, at least in cases in which a wounded human is able to report, the presence of consciousness to itself, which enables us in some way to enter into relationship with our very disability.[27]

Reflexive awareness illuminates our entire presence to the world. It transforms the ways we desire. It infiltrates our passions and needs. It recasts our behaviors as moral expression. Our appetites and wants, when personalized, become expansive and open-ended, experienced as dynamisms toward anything desirable in the world—but now known self-consciously. Such dynamisms are central to the phenomena of will and autonomy that make possible a certain freedom in our choices. Conscious reflexivity enables the person to take a stance in self-conscious relationship to desire. It makes possible—to the extent that my knowledge of myself, my history, my endowments, my compulsions are made self-consciously available—increasing degrees of limited self-possession. This personal ownership is based on the knowledge of who and what I am. It is an affirmation of who and what I am. It is a declaration of personal independence.

There is, then, no possibility for human agency without embodied awareness of awareness. There could be no questions, no question of ethics, without embodied A2—which is the human person. There would be no subjectivity. There would be no committed relationship. There would be no responsibility and freedom. There would be no self-accountable actions in space and time without personally endowed life-careers. There would be no ethical act (such action presupposes self knowledge and accountability for such knowledge), no ethical theory (theory is nothing other than an individual or corporate self-reflective systematization of human action).

Embodied awareness of awareness is what the human person is. As "embodied," we are animals—organic, developing, individual careers. As endowed with reflexive consciousness, we are personalized animals. Although there may be many workable definitions of what a human person is, I propose that the term "human person," applied to myself, is the entire individual career. The person, John Kavanaugh—the "self" or "I" he primarily refers to when he says these words—started when his individual life started ("I was born in 1941"; "I think I was conceived in springtime"), not when he started *thinking* about himself, or acquired mental states, or even *realized* he was a self, psychologically speaking.

To be a human person is to be inseparable from the facticity of body. To be a human person is to abide in time and history. A human person is unthinkable, unimaginable, without the endowment of reflexive consciousness that makes possible not just bodies but personal embodiment.

This chapter, like the following chapter, may seem rather remote from ethics—not to mention the ethics of killing. It is crucial, however, not only in understanding why there is ethics and why ethics is itself an implicit affirmation of our personhood but also in understanding what a human person is and is not. A human person is not a brain, nor the contents of a brain. A human person is an integrated, embodied life—among whose endowments is, after some maturation, a brain. Likewise, a human person is not some pure consciousness or spirit or intellect but a special kind of animal. We are personal animals because among our endowments is the capacity for awareness of our own act of awareness that makes us animals who are not only living a life but having a moral life.

4

Endowments of Embodied Persons

You can't equate the pig with the anencephalic infant. The anencephalic child is not the subject of life in any meaningful sense. That is to say, it does not possess that constellation of attributes— sense of self-awareness, anticipation of the future, memory of the past—that we have been discussing. The pig is clearly the subject of a meaningful life.

Gary Francione
Professor of Law, University of Pennsylvania[1]

Article 1. All human beings are born free and equal in dignity and rights. They are endowed with reason and conscience and should act towards one another in a spirit of brotherhood.

Universal Declaration of Human Rights[2]

The higher a nature the more intimate what comes from it, for its inwardness of activity corresponds to its rank in being. Inanimate bodies hold the lowest place of all; from them nothing comes save by the action of another.

Plants are higher; already in them there is an issuing from within. . . . Here the first degree of life may be discerned, for living things are those that set themselves into activity, whereas things that are in motion only inasmuch as they are acted on from outside are lifeless. Above plants there is a higher grade of life, that namely of sensitive things. Their proper process, though initiated from without, terminates within; the more developed the process, the more intimate this result. A sensible object impresses a form on the external senses, this goes into the imagination and then deeper into the store of memory. What begins from without is thus worked up within, for the sensitive powers are conscious within themselves. . . .

The supreme and perfect grade of life is found in mind, which can reflect on itself and understand itself. . . . The human intellect, though able to know itself, must start from outside objects and cannot know these without sense images. A more perfect intellectual life is that of pure spirits, where the mind does not proceed by introspection from outside things to know itself, but knows itself by itself.

Thomas Aquinas[3]

PERSONAL FOUNDATIONS

I have claimed that "embodied awareness of awareness," the description of human personhood, gives ethics its very meaning and makes ethics possible. To make such a claim is to offer one way of returning human persons to the center of ethical discourse.

This "centering" on the person may strike some academicians as "creeping foundationalism," a hankering after some indubitable and impregnable starting point. It is foundational, but it is only as invulnerable and indubitable as our fragile humanness itself. After all, even the most relentless deconstructionists and relativists posit their claims out of their lived experience as humans, and nothing else. Surely they would not be so other-worldly as to assert otherwise. To ground ethics in the human person, as I have been doing, is also to claim that each human being, as an embodied awareness-of-awareness, is constituted in a way that is peculiar to personalized bodies, capable of ethics. Each person is endowed with capacities that mark persons *as* persons.

A discussion of these endowments is crucial to philosophical ethics. They are the capacities that make ethics possible. They also are central to most moral disagreements concerning the taking of life. What kinds of beings *count* as persons? What is it about persons that leads us to make claims about their dignity and their rights? How do we determine the point when such a being begins and ends its career as a person?

The Universal Declaration of Human Rights boldly announces that human beings are "endowed" from their earliest moments with inherent properties that cannot be taken away from them. Yet a professor of law at the University of Pennsylvania Law School proclaims that a pig is the subject of a meaningful life, whereas a damaged human infant is not. Upon what evidence and with what criteria is such a judgment made? If one is indeed morally concerned about the treatment of animals, might not a brain-damaged newborn human deserve at least the care one would bestow on mice? This is only one of the common puzzles in contemporary debates about human identity and human rights. It is a result of, among other things, deep confusion over what constitutes human personhood.

Thus, I have begun this investigation into philosophical ethics with an initial consideration of the meaning of human personhood. Such an investigation of embodied self-consciousness and its endowments is not entirely new. As we have seen, it is congruent with the work of phenomenologists, personalists, and some existentialists; it also is indirectly related to the theories of Thomas Aquinas.

Obviously, Aquinas's own writings did not face the challenge—nor reap the benefit—of modern science; of Descartes' radical move toward subjectivity; of Hume's skepticism; of Kant's transcendental method; of the great suspicions in Nietzsche, Marx, and Freud; of the Anglo-American linguistic turn; or of the present cynicism concerning traditional philosophical questions. Moreover, Aquinas's positions are not widely examined today quite possibly out of wariness about any notions of "substance," "nature," and "teleology." Such wariness is warranted, especially if the only notions of substance and nature are freighted with baggage piled on by Descartes and Hume. This is not to say that Descartes and Hume were wholly mistaken in their positions. It is only to suggest that philosophy did not begin with them and to point out the fact that "postmodernism" is precisely that: *post*-modernity.

What if postmodernists rediscovered *pre*modernity? What if they found out that, in rebelling against the "modern" models of humanness constructed by Descartes, Hume, Locke, and Kant, they were not automatically forced to announce the "end of man" but only the end of a pretentious substitute? Notions such as "substance" and "nature" need not be construed the way most contemporaries presume. In fact, Aquinas used these tools to describe human reality. His use of these tools is utterly unlike anything found in Descartes, Kant, or the British empiricists.[4]

We humans are integrated and unified entities (substances) and members of a class of entities that share common, species-exclusive endowments (nature). In other words, I am a substance participating in a class of beings with specific capacities that (in our case) are the conditions for embodiment. This is not an "eternal" substance or "ahistorical" nature. It is simply a way of talking about what it is to be a human rather than something else.

An embodied, self-conscious being is given to himself or herself as constituted with the capacities that being bodied and self-conscious require. I experience my own capacities to receive information about myself and the world in a complex process of external sensation. I integrate, process, store, and recall this highly localizable information in the cerebral cortex. I also am quite clearly responsive to the world I experience, through an impressive range of affective capacities. Aristotle and Aquinas understood this process of information-gathering and responsiveness, in their own limited ways, as sensation (external and internal) and appetite (dynamisms toward sense-known desirable objects). On this level of information and appetite, we probably share the processes of learning and responsiveness with nonpersonal animals. One could even say that there are analogous processes of information intake and response in mechanical computational systems.[5] More significantly, however, I experience myself as endowed with a reflexively conscious capacity to stand in relationship to my own experience. This capacity to act with concomitant awareness characterizes my engagement as free; this capacity does not seem to be shared by animals that are not human—even in their most mature and highly developed states.

I encounter the world as an open and flexible experience. Such encounters contrast with other moments when my actions may be more automatic, even driven—forced or blindly necessitated. The world and my experience of it is a problem to me. It also may be a mystery. There is a depth to my encounter with the world because of the self-reflexive consciousness that marks it. Thus Aquinas, in the passage at the head of this chapter, characterizes the human engagement of the world as being of greatest *intimacy*: the Latin *intime*, meaning depth as well as interiority.[6] He asserts that any being that knows itself is capable of an intimacy far deeper than a being that does not know itself. He would find the anger or the love of any human more profoundly stirring than the anger or love of any nonhuman because of the depth of a consciousness that is conscious of itself in relating to me. No doubt there is great affective bonding between humans and animals—but it is not between selves. That is the very reason it is so much easier to relate to one's dog, for example, than one's spouse or friend: The dog has no ego to interfere with one's own.

One of the reasons for my experiential depth is that I am able to relate myself to my own experience. This relationship is the key not only to freely given intimacies but to moral responsibility. The personal moral question—What am I to do?—emerges only because of the fact that I need not act in any predetermined way.

This question of action results from my engagement with the world in an open manner—not fixed, not rigidly programmed, not always impulsive. In fact, I am quite self-consciously aware of the startling difference in my responses when I experience myself as somehow driven, forced, or compelled. Coercion is indubitably different than the ordinarily deliberative and evaluative "distance" that I can entertain when I consider taking a course of action.

The endowment of reflexive consciousness "frees up" my responses to the world. They are not forced or compelled. They are not fixed by my history. Sometimes, in moments of great creativity or resistance, they are just the opposite. More ordinarily they are at least deliberate, expressive, and interpretative—which phenomena I will soon examine more closely.

Knowing the world as other than the I who knows it, I can assume a questioning and evaluative stance toward it and toward myself in responding to it. Thus, I relate to my actions as my own. I know them as of me and by me. When I act, I am not merely regurgitating internalized information. As a centered consciousness, I can make affirmations in and through them. My actions embody and express me—what I am, who I am. They are self-revelations. They reveal my personal reality, my self-consciously chosen intentions, my moral life. To the extent that I know them, own them, and express them as mine, they are given the quality of what I call personal morality.

An act enters the ethical realm only if it is reflexively known by the person who acts, is self-consciously owned by that person, and is self-consciously performed by that person. This emphasis on the self as the "one who acts," to be sure, does not alter the fact that we can only begin (as we have seen) as embodied: situated in space and time and inherently constituted by cultural, social, familial, and physical forces. I must emphasize that this is not a return to some solipsistic or isolated "self" that somehow sees itself in a mirror before encountering the lived world. It is, however, an insistence that ethical action would not be introduced into the world if there were no ethical agent endowed with the reflexive capacity for such agency.[7]

AWARENESS OF AWARENESS, SELVES, AND PERSONS

The endowment of reflexive consciousness (or awareness of awareness) presents a particular quandary. It has never been measured, observed, or quantified. It has only been engaged—in human experiences. This quandary has caused problems not only for Hume—who could never find the self in observations or perceptions—and for Skinner, who rejects its possibility because it cannot be scientifically calibrated; it also is troubling for most people of modern scientific consciousness.

Walker Percy retells the story of Sir John Eccles lecturing at Harvard about the human brain. The brilliant neuroscientist ended his presentation with the contention that, although the brain indeed was explicable in terms of evolution and physical chemistry, the human endowment of consciousness was not. Its source must somehow be transcendent—at least to the brain. There was hissing in the audience.[8]

This account is curiously similar to an incident that occurred at the university where I received my doctorate. Eccles was greeted with great resistance (especially from the philosophers of science) when he stated that all of his years of clinical medicine and research on the brain led him to the conclusion that human self-consciousness could not be exhaustively explained in material categories. To the numbed questioner who asked how such a nonmaterial phenomenon could possibly exist, Eccles simply stated that we must not begin with any other presuppositions than who and what we are and do. We have self-consciousness. Our lived conviction about its existence is a necessary condition not only for science but for culture, artistic expression, and philosophy. If we cannot explain self-consciousness in terms of material categories, we need not conclude that self-consciousness does not exist. Our material categories simply are inadequate to explain it. The map that guides us in human understanding is too small, too narrow, too selective.

Colin McGinn in *The Mysterious Flame* writes tellingly of the illusiveness of consciousness: "Where does it come from? What manner of secretion is this? How does mere meat turn itself into conscious awareness . . . there must be some kind of natural process behind this astonishing leap, but this process is obscure."[9] McGinn is convinced of the underlying unity in the "mind-brain link," although he suspects an irreducible difference in the faculties by which we might know them. "Why should everything that exists be similar to objects in perceived space . . . ?

We are trying to crack open the nut of consciousness with tools derived from perception of the physical world and the structure of language, but it is not surprising that these tools will not do the job."[10] Although he thinks there is likely an intractable mystery in consciousness (what I would prefer to call reflexive consciousness), he nonetheless rejects any suggestion of dualism, supernaturalism, or other mystification. Rightly so, because he identifies such mystifications with substance dualism that entails a disembodied consciousness from a parallel world. Many philosophers and scientists share this position, if they are willing to acknowledge the inescapable reality of consciousness. Unlike those who simply deny that consciousness is real or reduce it to elementary blind neural interactions, they propose the "mysterious flame" solution or hope for some eventual solution.[11]

I entertain a third way: one personal organic unity that is an embodied, reflexively conscious career. It is not my brain or my awareness of awareness that knows; it is *I* who know, endowed with brainy and self-conscious capacities. Among the endowments of this unity is one that, at least as far as we now know, is inexplicable in sheer material, quantitative terms. Could it be possible that the reason A2 cannot be explained materially is the fact that it is not a material endowment, although the development and processing of the brain is required for its embodied *actuation?* If we examine this reflexive act of consciousness, such a possibility suggests itself.

Awareness of awareness is an act wholly present to itself. It is the "bending back" of consciousness upon itself—an act not like that of seeing oneself in a mirror but of seeing oneself behind oneself and in front of oneself at the same time. In this total return of awareness upon itself, it covers itself fully and transparently. Notice: We are not speaking of the content of consciousness, nor are we speaking of the "self," which obviously has no such total reflexivity. Nor are we speaking to the habit of having a "reflective life." There obviously are moments when we are more or less reflective—or not at all. *Reflexive consciousness,* it seems, is always "on," at least in the sense that I am aware of being aware even when I am not attending to the fact.

Awareness of awareness is an act, an acting, which is both knowing and known at the same time—fully subjective, but having itself as a concomitant object in the experience of other objects. If it were material, it would have to be in two places, wholly and entire, at the same time. There may be some quantum explanation of this phenomenon, or a modularity in the brain that gives the illusion of unity, or an astounding number of computations in the cortex that gives us the feel of reflexivity; in the absence of compelling evidence, however, concluding that there is something about our cognitive endowments that is not exhaustively explained by or reduced to the organicity of a brain is provisionally warranted.

Could this be why some philosophers declare reflexive consciousness to be nonexistent? Obviously it cannot be found on a map that handles only material coordinates. Because it has no "place in the brain," it is nowhere. Because it has no location, it is no material thing. Does that mean that it is nothing, however? Could it be an act, a something, an endowment that is nonmaterial?

Material objects are extended, ranging over space and time, having parts contiguous to and outside of other parts. Material objects can be "present" to or cover other material or even parts of themselves. Thus, the eye can be present to the object as colored, but the eye is not present to the eye: The eye does not see itself seeing. The hand can cover the other hand or even fold in half upon itself, but it cannot stay where it is and cover itself. To approximate the full kind of reflexivity experienced in awareness of awareness, the hand would have to stay put and get around and behind itself at the same time. Because it is extended in space, it cannot remain in place and cover itself as a whole, without losing its previous place.

In awareness of awareness, in consciousness of consciousness under the conditions of my own embodiment, I experience this phenomenon. In awareness of awareness, the act covers, converges upon itself. It is not spatial, it is not made up of quantifiable parts. In this sense, it is nonmaterial.

If such a rendering of the "nonmateriality" of A2 is adequate and accurate as a confirmation of Eccles' position concerning human self-consciousness, then there is indeed something about human knowing, human freedom, human covenants, human beings that is not reducible to space and time.

Because A2 is a nonmaterial human endowment, it is not *in itself* determined by environment, by the brain, by input, by physical evolutionary laws. The human, however—an *embodied* awareness-of-awareness—is. Personal animals actualize their endowments only in the context of space and history, subject to all the determinants, historical causes, and social constituents that a human body must have. Embodiment is the historical-spatial occasion and locality of self-conscious human action.

When my body is damaged, when my brain is injured, *I* am injured. The *human person* is damaged. When my historical conditions change or if my social context were other than it is, I indeed am profoundly affected. What remains throughout the variables of cultures, what is *not* intrinsically affected by traditions, what is *not* given to me by social arrangements, what is *not* bestowed upon me by language or intersubjectivity, however, is my endowment of reflexive consciousness.

A person, a human self, is a totality. A human person is spread out in space and history; subject to development; formed by information of environment, genetic code, molecular chemistry, and historical accident. The personal self is the whole career—generated, elaborated, and realized over a finite and individual time frame. For embodied persons, these determinants are the necessary conditions of historical actuality—from which we, as embodied, have never been separated.

The endowment of reflexive consciousness that is at the heart of self-discovery, self-interpretation, and self-expression becomes—perhaps surprisingly—the radical basis of human equality. Because it is a nonmaterial endowment, no cultural, political, or biological condition lessens it. It also is the capacity that makes us personally unique in this individuated capacity for self-defining action in ethical choice. Only I have the capacity to possess myself and express that self-possession in moral action. Herein, I am irreplaceable in the moral sense. Herein as well, however, you are as irreplaceable and unique as I am. We are radically equal.

THE ENDOWMENT OF FREEDOM

To be endowed with the capacity for freedom is to be open to self-ownership. That power need not ever be exercised, but it is an inherent capacity in any embodied self-conscious person.

For those who have either a dualistic or a reductionistic view of human reality, the existence of such a power in humans is troubling. If one holds to the "split off" world of disembodied mind, human freedom cannot be engaged in space and time because the ahistorical self is presumed to be unconditioned by space and time. Thus, for a philosopher such as Sartre, freedom becomes a phenomenon of pure negation that can have no concrete actuality or limiting definition. Sartre's radical subjectivity ultimately is cut off from local or historical significance.[12]

If one holds material reductionism, on the other hand, brute structures of time and place dictate the drama of human action. There is no need—indeed, no room—for self-conscious agency. The behaviorism of B. F. Skinner, for example, begins with a presumption that "freedom" (if there could even be such a strange thing) must somehow be outside the realm of history and oddly immune from causes, purposes, and reasons.

This presumption preempts even the possibility of a free act of an embodied-freedom. According to the presuppositions of Skinner, any free act must somehow be uncaused, unmotivated, and unreasoned. After all, if there is a cause or motive to our behavior, it is the cause or motive that moves us, not our "freedom." Skinner's *presumed* concept of freedom is wholly ahistorical, atemporal, disembodied. That is why it *cannot* exist for him.

Yet Skinner finds himself in strange, almost perverse, agreement with his well-known opposite, Sartre. Oddly enough, they share the presupposition of a world split between pure consciousness and pure historical and spatial structure. Sartre lives with the dualism because, for him, the data of human consciousnesses are inescapable, self-evident, and irrefutable. The consciousness or awareness of a cause or motive is precisely the negation of the cause's supremacy in one's life. Skinner rejects the dualism, however, because the requirements of concomitant consciousness are—to a dogmatic materialism—incomprehensible.[13]

For one who acknowledges the primordial human encounter of the world as an embodied self-consciousness, however, something is experienced that might be called human freedom.

Consider, for example, a young girl who is afraid of heights. She is twelve, and she is not even self-consciously aware of the fact that she fears high places. She simply stays away from them, sometimes not even knowing that she stays away. She might explain her behaviors by saying, "I just don't like it. It's a drag."

Most of us know that we have engaged in behaviors or had attitudes that we didn't even know we were involved in. Some liars are most adept when they don't realize they are lying. Some of our depressions can be most debilitating before we even know we have them. The alcoholic who doesn't suspect he is, is most caught. People who are most unaware of their prejudices are most prejudiced.

At fourteen, our young eighth-grade graduate is forced onto a Ferris wheel by a group of boys who have suspected that behind her bravado was fear. They do not realize it was terror. Yet that is what it becomes for her, when they force her onto the amusement park ride: She is so intensely traumatized that the machine must be stopped. Now she *knows*, as she never did, that she is afraid. At this stage, with this new awareness, she manages her life more efficiently and honestly. She just stays away from high places: She plans her schooling, orchestrates her dates, chooses her friends, opts for entertainment with her newly accepted knowledge in mind.

We know that when we become self-consciously aware of a pattern of behavior or mood, we can manage the environment with that awareness in mind. Such coping is paltry, to be sure. Nevertheless, this reality is different than our earliest stage.

At sixteen, the young woman meets someone who is enamored of planes and mountain climbing (which she discovers only after months of growing to know and like him considerably). When she finds out and reveals her own fears to him, he makes no effort to change her. He does ask her why, however. He asks only that she try to understand—for his sake—why she has such a gnawing fear of something he so fully enjoys. She goes through therapy. She discovers that her fear is rooted in a childhood trauma: She was left alone in a tree by her older brother, who abandoned her to play baseball. He warned her never to tell anyone.

At seventeen, then, she not only knows that she is afraid; she knows why. Although this deeper level of self-knowledge, of self-intimacy, which is made possible by reflexive consciousness, does not change the fact of her fear, it does disarm the fear.

At eighteen, knowing that she is afraid of heights—and knowing why she is afraid—she makes her first small attempts at entering the fear. By the end of the year, she is willing to fly. She finds it a thrill. The thrill is not only in the fact of flying, in being with her friend in his delight, but also in continuing to bear the now-lightened burden of a disarmed fear that will always be a part of her, yet will not dominate her.

Many things may have happened to her over these years, and there are many ways to describe them. One of the things that has happened, however, can be called an experienced process of embodied freedom. It is a movement of increasing self-understanding: a reflexive consciousness of the conditions of one's history, context, motives, capacities, and influences.

Reflexive consciousness does not obliterate the past; it brings the past into self-conscious remembrance. It does not cancel what Freud calls the unconscious; as a force of liberation, it brings it into appropriated awareness. Reflexive consciousness is the essential requirement for meeting Freud's goal of bringing human "itness" into the realm of the "I."[14] A reflexive awareness of motives and causes is not in itself a further motive or cause—unless one sees it as the inherent causality made possible by the fact of our being human.

In the sense, then, Sartre was right: As human, we are indeed condemned, determined—but to be free. We are structured, constituted, as free beings—beings capable of self-conscious relationship with our past and our own structure. We cannot escape that fact. That is what exercising our personhood means. The crucial defining determinant of our lived reality is the fact that we can freely engage our own identity as well as the external forces that form us.

The entire process is characterized by greater self-knowledge and increasing self-ownership. In the young woman's very act of becoming aware of her fear and why it is present, it owns her less as she comes to possess herself more. This process is a movement of increasing self-definition and self-donation. She is able to give herself more of herself as she comes to know herself more fully.

This is not the experience of a pure consciousness that is utterly disengaged from the structures of space and time. In fact, the structures of space and time, which in many ways own and define her, become the very occasions for her increasing knowledge and owning of her self. It is a limited, human, bodied freedom. Thus, Merleau-Ponty in *Phenomenology of Perception* reminds us that our freedom is just the opposite of some ahistorical and acausal being: Historical causality actually is the occasion for a freedom that is human.

> All explanations of my conduct in terms of my past, my temperament and my environment are therefore true, provided that they may be regarded not as separable contributions, but as moments of my total being. . . . I am a psychological and historical structure, and have received, with existence, a manner of existing, a style. All my actions and thoughts stand in a relationship to this structure, and even a philosopher's thought is merely a way of making explicit his hold on the world, and what he is. The fact remains that I am free, not in spite of, or in the hither side of, these motivations, but by means of them. For this significant life, this

certain significance of nature and history which I am, does not limit my access to the world, but on the contrary is my means of entering into communication with it.[15]

The freedom of a human person is a freedom that is an *endowment* of *embodied* awareness of awareness. It is the only freedom with which a human person is capacitated. Through this endowment, we have potentialities to grow in self-possession, to define ourselves more fully through actions we call "moral," and to give ourselves away more profoundly.

THE ENDOWMENT OF LOVE IN SELF-CONSCIOUS AFFIRMATION

Our ability to enter into a reflexively conscious relationship with the world is a capacity for affirmation. It is the ability to say "yes" as well as "no." It is the ability to take ownership of our responses to the world. Our engagement with the world is not automatic. Our acceptance of the world and ourselves is not reactive or mechanical. We need not bestow our "yes" upon the world. We need not love it.

This phenomenon is more primary than language. Language—not mere communication or signaling—is at its propositional core an affirmation of and by the speaker. Language entails "saying" something, expressing and intending it. To speak is to have something to say that is mine. It is not the mere formulation of a sentence; it is the declaration of one who declares, who judges and affirms.

Mere sentences are regurgitations. Machines often can fire them out more effectively than humans. A sentence that is an *affirmation* by the speaker, a *revelation* of the speaker's self-conscious capacity to take a stance toward the input received, however, is the revelation of personal reality, the embodiment of human intent. Human language is not only a revelation of the cues and signals that a human has received; it is the unveiling of a self-possessed response to the world.

Similarly, the use of "concepts" is not the key to understanding human experience in the world. It is not even the linchpin that holds together our humanity in a way that is unique to us. Even machines muster analogues of conceptualization. At the heart of the concept, humanly understood, is the *affirmation* of the concept, the *ownership* of it. This is behind the irrepressible cascade of concept-affirmations in every two-year-old. They are all saying, "yes!" in naming.

When Helen Keller writes in *The Story of My Life* of her childhood breakthrough into language and concept, central in her realization is that she can enter into a self-conscious relationship with the buzzing phantasmagoria of cues and signals that were seemingly invading her life. The breakthrough is the ownership of the cues in the concept of "water." She is driven by the sheer delight at engaging this capacity to run through the house and the farmland affirming in concept: *water.* She is saying, "I am saying this." Keller had experienced her "I" before this time—and she felt the imprisonment of it through the deficits of deafness and blindness. What she discovered, with the help of Annie Sullivan, was that she could affirm that "I" in language and express it through concept.[16]

The uttering of affirmation is a "yes" to the world as it is a "yes" to one's self as a center of experience. It is a "yes" to one's personhood discovered, of one's freedom—not coerced but invited. I propose that this affirmation of the being of who and what we are is love. It is not mere acceptance. It is not resignation or passivity before the givenness of ourselves and our world. It is the self-conscious appropriation and affirmation of our reality.

By the fact of our personhood, our self-conscious embodiment, we can freely affirm and love ourselves, the world, and the other. We need not, however. As opposed to any other being that is merely receptive and ultimately passive before the world and its impact, we are not forced to be who and what we are. Because we can say yes, we can say no. When you and I ask of ourselves, "Will I, ought I, should I?" we are entering the realm of ethics by the endowment of our personhood.

In contrast to the uniqueness of any material object, living organism, or sensate animal, materially actual in its own space and time, you and I can actualize ourselves in the stance and attitude that we self-consciously affirm. Therefore each of us, so endowed, is morally, ethically unique. No one can possibly take my place in saying my own "yes" to existence. No one else can place my act of love. Yet each person has the *endowment* to do so. None of us can be replaced in this regard, but each of us, so endowed, is bonded in radical unity and equality with the other.

No one of us is greater than any other in terms of our *endowments* as persons. Some of us may be further developed in our fulfillments, organic or otherwise. Some of us may be more mature or supple. Some of us may be more greatly gifted by the contingencies of time and place, genetic endowment, physical nutriment, cultural expanse. Each and all of us, however, are radically equal and unique in our capacity to say our own "yes"—even if it might not ever get spoken. The child with Down's syndrome might say his "yes." The socially inept savant may say hers. Geniuses may say their own as well. Whenever a human career begins, the latent capacity for love is present. The contingencies of time, place, and structure determine only whether and how that power to love is actualized.

ENDOWED HUMAN PERSONS

The human person is an embodied, self-conscious drama. We are life stories, narratives that start with endowments that make possible our becoming aware of our own stories and eventually writing our own autobiographies within the limits of our diverse histories.

There may be other persons that are not human. They might have other embodiments or no embodiment at all. If nonhuman animals, for example, are discovered to have reflexive consciousness, and thereby embodied self-consciousness, they would be persons—even if not of the human variety—and it would be appropriate to treat them as self-knowing and self-possessing beings. There might be all kinds of self-conscious beings that have no historical career. This account, then, is not at all speciesist. It is personalist. Thus, Colin McGinn's argument—which he correctly associates with the positions of Peter Singer and Evelyn Pluhar—that personal dignity must be denied, on homocentric grounds, to extra-terrestrials, God, Jesus, or animals that *have* awareness of awareness is incorrect. The issue is the endowment of reflexive awareness.[17]

The use of the word *person* to describe our human situation of embodiment is related to its earliest origins. The Latin *persona* (*per sonans*: speaking or sounding through), which is related to the Greek *prosopon* (*pros opon*: see through and out) was used to indicate the mask worn by actors in a drama. To be a person is to be an expressive animal, a self-creating drama, a center of action, a narrative becoming conscious of itself, revealing and yet concealed through the embodiment of mask. The mask is not a pretense—although it can be. It is a revelation, an expression, an externalization that is one with the actor.

Human persons, as embodied careers, are creatures of time. We unfold and develop. Each one of us is a career-totality, not summed up at any given moment or place, not reducible to our beginnings or our end. We are, each of us, the entire drama from beginning to end.

Whenever an individual career begins—whenever the process of unfolding, developing, and revealing begins—a human person begins. Whenever the career, the life story, is definitively over, a human person ends. Determining those points of beginning and ending will be crucial when we ask what actions are proper with respect to the intended negation of a human person's life.

We can call the human person, in this sense, a *historical and natural* self; although this usage would not be the most common sociological or psychological one. The self who writes this book—his gender, his color-blindness, his genetic propensities, his reflexive consciousness (even before he had primary and secondary sex characteristics, complete eyes, a weak lumbar region, or a functioning cortex)—began when his life-career, his story began. That same self will end when he comes irreversibly to an end. This notion is quite different from the concept of the self or the person as an "active conscious subject" (which was somehow stuck on a human body when brain states occurred) or a function of social recognition and interaction.[18] The choice of such criteria certainly is an option, but it is important to know the differences and the implications. On the account offered here, the personal reality of John Kavanaugh started before, and is the condition for, all activities of consciousness or interpersonal encounter.

The personal self is not some hidden, transcendental "core" that is "behind" all human agency. It is the totality of a human career, generated out of and into local determinants, developing in a concrete place and time, falling short of or achieving fulfillments of uniquely individual and commonly shared capacities. One of these capacities—awareness of awareness—enables the human career to be a self-conscious one, so that all the behaviors and processes of the career can become expressions and embodiments. Like all of my capacities or endowments, A2 was and is *of* me, this unique career, from the moment I started.

The development of the personal self is profoundly influenced and modified by all of the contingencies of time and place: not only that I was conceived by two humans who carried my genetic capacities; not only that I developed fetally without major assault or trauma; not only that I had enough oxygen and sustenance upon birth; not only that I was cared for and socialized by loving persons—but also by the fact that I happened to be at a certain corner in a certain moment and bumped into someone who would be a friend to me all my life and modify my own understanding of my self and my world. The human self is not some isolated consciousness over and against culture or intersubjectivity or sociality; it is enfleshed only and through these very determinants.

At this point, some readers might suspect an "ontological turn" away from previous phenomenological reflection. They are right. Such a turn to the ontological structure of human reality is required, ultimately, of any answer to the question, "What am I?"

Boethius' famous definition of the person as "an individual substance of a rational nature" [19] is not unconnected with the notion of *person* I have been discussing—although his emerges from a profoundly different tradition, strongly grounded in ontological commitments that are not commonly shared today.

Boethius' first characteristic of the person is *individuality*. As person, I am individual—a being in some significant ways on my own, in myself, rather than inhering in another. My capacities and activities are *of* and *in* me. My brain is part of me; I am not part of my brain. Although I am not in isolation or in solitary independence from others, I still experience my own given situation as mine. I have my own dynamic processes that are of and for me, my own purposes, my own tendency toward the fulfillment of my capacities and potentialities. As embodied self-consciousness, I experience these activities in such unity and concert that their "dislocation" and fragmentation disorient and startle me.

This emphasis on "individual" might be misunderstood in some atomistic sense—that I am somehow so radically "my own" that I am separated from conditions of history and society that quite clearly, as embodied, actually are part of the constitution of who and what I am. I suspect that Boethius, and certainly Aquinas, did not mean "individual" in this sense. Most assuredly I do not.

To say that I am a "substance" is to say that I am an internal unity—again emphasizing that I am a being in itself and not a mere appendage to another. I have my own intrinsic organizing principle, integrating all of my activities in concert for the good of myself as one organism. This conception does not deny that I have dependencies on larger systems or on other beings like myself. It is only a naming of the fact that I am, in a significant way, a unity—a living, substantial unity.

Although dangers lurk in such a notion—the danger of presumed mere "objectness" and staticity as well as the danger that one might conceive one's substantialness as some kind of underlying pin-cushion to which accidental attributes are stuck on and in—it offers some service. The reality of myself does perdure through time and alteration, even if I undergo massive damage. It is "poor John" who is so damaged. Even if I say that I am a "different man" than I was twenty years ago, it is I who say it and make the connection, presupposing an even greater underlying continuity.

The person is the totality, the unity developing through all the stages of personhood, over the vicissitudes of change and chance and choice. If I change with respect to my "substantial" identity, then "I" am no more.

Although the word *nature* is troubling to some thinkers, it actually can be quite simple and serviceable.[20] We can use it to refer to the fact that there are different *kinds* of individuals in the world, differentiated according to the kinds of activities they and only they are capable of exercising. Nature, in this sense, is simply the answer to the question, What kind of reality are you?—answered from the point of view of the kinds of capacities-to-act that I share with other individuals of my class and seem not to share with others. Thus, it is a very dynamic term; the complaint that *nature* is too rigid and fixed a notion to be helpful any longer is merely an indication that it has been misunderstood or too constricted in its application.[21] This use of *nature* is central to Aquinas' notion of "natural law." It does not mean the "brute state of nature," or "mother nature," or "doing what comes naturally." It means, at its core, a fidelity to who and what I am, a personal nature, with certain shared capacities and traits common to my kind.

Rationality—one of those hallmark capacities—is a term meant to loosen any supposed rigidity in the definition of nature as it is applied to human persons. Boethius uses it to specify what kind of nature we have. We are of that class of beings who are capacitated with reason, an endowment whereby we exercise intellectual knowledge of the world and engage it accordingly. I would have no quarrels with this emphasis on rationality if it were taken to mean the endowment of reflexive consciousness. Too often, however, rationality is equated with mere technical expertise, or the potential for language or tool-making, or the power of abstract conceptualization or various other sundry activities—most of which have for their condition the reflexive consciousness I discussed in Chapter 3.

Another difficulty with the qualification of our human nature as "rational" is the mistaken tendency to isolate reason in human experience. If we can understand that rationality is inseparable from all other parts of our experience, it would be quite properly effective in distinguishing our nature from any other kind of nature. We would be taking note of the fact that reason transforms and is transformed by affect, emotion, and embodiment and that it is not, in isolation, the qualifying characteristic of our personhood.

The dangers of dualism and rationalism are as persistent as they are treacherous. Thus, my preferred employment of "embodied consciousness-of-consciousness," with both parts of the term mutually constituting and modifying the other, may well be less open to misinterpretation.

PERSONAL NATURE

To speak of a human as a personal nature is to refer to the fact of embodiment. The human cannot be reduced to some rigid or fixed model of nature. A human—paradoxically because of the "natural" endowment of self-consciousness—transcends any attempt to fully constrain human behavior.[22] We humans, as personal animals, share an "open" nature because "what" we are is the kind of being endowed with distinguishing capacities of *self-conscious* embodiment whereby we are freed from any inflexible or determined "playing out" of our natural drives. We are not "owned by" our in-built capacities because one of our capacities is an endowment wherein we can own ourselves.[23]

We do not play out some fixed script. We become actors, agents, because part of the scripting and constitution of our personhood is our capacity to own our roles and create much of the script. This capacity, as we shall see, is really what our ethical life is all about.

We *discover* the "nature" of a being by looking at what it does. Thus, we can say, "That is the kind of being that does X, Y, and Z." Observation, even of ourselves, is the only way we can begin. Thus, our reflections on embodied self-consciousness have been based on our embodied revelations as well as our consciousness of our own consciousness as it is acting. A human being is a kind of being with capacities to act in embodied, self-conscious ways. We conclude that we have such a nature by observing what we and others do. Because we observe that we act in certain ways, we know that we have the capacity or endowment to act in those ways; therefore we conclude that we are the "kind" of being so endowed.[24]

That is the *logic of discovery*. It is not the *logic of existential reality*, however. Existentially, there are different kinds, different "natures," capacitated to act and interact in the world differently. These capacities can be actualized or discovered or identified as unique traits.

The only way I can get to know you, to understand who and what you are, is to observe in some way your revelatory actions. My observation of your actions does not bestow upon you your capacity to act, however. You can act whether I know it or not. My inability to observe that you are capable of love is not necessarily a revelation of whether you have that capacity or not; it is only a revelation about the extent of my observations.

Thus, whether I approach your personal identity through the mediation of "activities" "text," social role, communication theory, or semiotics—and I must make these as well as other entries into my discovery of you—all of these are of *you* as writer, agent, communicator, symbolizer.

My observations of you, my discovery of you, does not make you what you are. It only makes my knowledge of you what it is. You act not because I acknowledge it but because you are inherently endowed for such actions. You are who and what you are—a self-conscious embodied career—whether I observe it or not and whether you reveal it or not, whether you perform it or not. For although I *discover* the world and myself by a process of observing actions, moving to endowments and then to kinds or natures, in reality the relationship is different.

There are different kinds of beings. They are different because they have different capacities and endowments that are open to activation. Capacities need not be activated or realized or fulfilled. Endowments need not be exercised or engaged. In controversies of medical ethics, consequently, if one holds to an endowment theory rather than a performance theory, a handicapped or undeveloped or "vegetative" human is an endowed human person, not some other kind of being.

Human infants do not become persons when they start thinking they are persons. Thinking is just one stage of personal development, made possible by the capacity to do so. A woman in a sixteen-year coma does not cease being a human person and then suddenly have her personhood stuck back on when she revives. She was never in a vegetative "state." She was in the state of being a human person, endowed with human capacities and yet so massively damaged in the cortex that many of these capacities could not be exercised, few of them could be revealed, and for a while none could be externally acknowledged by others. What she regains upon revival are the organic conditions required for the embodied self-expression of these capacities.[25]

Finally, with regard to the argument over animal rights that began this chapter: One most assuredly cannot "equate the pig with the anencephalic infant." The pig is of an entirely different class of living beings, and it is not endowed with the capacities that the damaged human child has. The damaged and not fully developed infant is a stage in a total human career, not a potential human or something inferior to a pig. The pig may be "better off" than the child. The pig may stunningly outperform the child. The pig may surely be more serviceable and useful. On the account offered in this chapter, however, the child is a human person with potentials. These potentials may or not be realized. The endowments—not the exercise or actualization of them— make the child a human person, however.

These claims are hotly contested by philosophers and activists in the animal rights movements. A recent example is Pluhar's *Beyond Prejudice: The Moral Significance of Human and Nonhuman Animals*. There are two pillars to Pluhar's thesis. First, persons are only those who have "full" personhood, or moral agency. They have *exhibited* the capacities for self-knowledge and responsibility that mark adult humans as moral agents. These, on Pluhar's account, are "full" persons. Second, in comparison to the way "marginal" humans behave, animals perform much more effectively and so should be given at least the same kind of treatment, protection, and respect that we give infants or brain-damaged humans who are not "full-fledged persons." Pluhar, impressed by the activities of monkeys and birds, writes, "Even primates considerably less well endowed mentally than chimps have demonstrated capacities beyond the abilities of some humans. . . . Birds can carry out acts that appear to require considerable planning, cooperation. . . . Unfortunately, there are many humans who could never equal any of these feats."[26]

Two problems (neither of which Pluhar addresses in the 360 pages of her book) demand attention, however. The first is this: Is personhood an ontological reality or a social construction? This question has been seductive for people interested in excluding others from the privileged status of "full" personhood. Human history is filled with attempts to bar certain humans from "full-fledged" personal status. The speculative Hegel and the practical Mill both had doubts about "wild aborigines." Marx suspected capitalists; capitalists wondered about the proletariat. Women in some countries still do not make the cut in qualifying for the "full-fledged" team. Fetuses are "tissue," criminals are "monsters," the enemy are "devils." If one becomes a person only by dictate of state, human fiat, performance, or achievement, our dignity and "human rights" are indeed figments of imagination. If personhood is an ontological and inalienable condition, however, our dignity, our rights, are real.

What I have proposed in this chapter is this: One is either a human person or not a human person. A human person is an unfolding reality, a historical being in which personal endowments make possible the emergence of activities, among which are knowing, loving, and choosing freely. Many humans never "fulfill" their potentials, whether through a lack of maturation or opportunity. Many others can no longer fulfill their potential because of trauma to or aging of the human body. They are still persons, however, even though unfulfilled or injured.

Pluhar does not consider this option because of a second fundamental mistake. She identifies personal reality with the *presence* of certain activities. Our actions, however, only *reveal* our personal nature; they do not *constitute* it.

Helen Keller was *what* she was—a human person with a human nature and human endowments—before she ever *performed* like one. What her tutor Annie Sullivan gave to her was neither human personhood nor her capacities but the opportunity to actualize and express them. If we do not perform well because of lack of development or education, we are unfulfilled persons—but persons nonetheless. If we are afflicted by Alzheimer's disease, we are not "marginal" persons but wounded ones.

Obviously, most chimpanzees and chicks perform more impressively than babies and comatose patients. The former are animals exhibiting and actualizing their endowments, often in admirable behavior. The latter, however, have personal endowments, albeit unrealized and unexpressed. We are far more than a stage of development, the achievements we win or the losses we suffer. That is what it means to be a human kind of being, rather than something else.

The human person is endowed with personal dignity by the fact of what a human person is: an embodied self-conscious career. This is the givenness of our being human. It is not given to us by state, environment, attribution of others, bonding, or the privilege of class—although these factors are all constitutive of the manner in which my career as a person is elaborated and actualized. A person is a person, whether unrecognized or unwanted, legitimated by law, deficient by organic damage, undeveloped by reason of temporality, or unrealized in potentialities because of historical conditions.

The dignity of the human person resides in the capacities with which such personhood is endowed: the capacity for self-consciousness, the capacity for freedom, and the capacity for the affirmation of love. These endowments characterize that kind of being called human. As members of a kind, humans partake in a nature. That nature is personal, however. For that reason, it is a free nature. It is a morally charged one.

5

Personal Entries into Ethics

If adversity and hopeless sorrow have completely taken away the relish for life; if the unfortunate one, strong in mind, indignant at his fate rather than desponding or dejected, wishes for death, and yet preserves his life without loving it—not from inclination or fear, but from duty— then his maxim has a moral worth.

Immanuel Kant[1]

He who saves a fellow creature from drowning does what is morally right, whether his motive be duty, or the hope of being paid for his trouble; he who betrays the friend that trusts him, is guilty of a crime, even if his object be to serve another friend to whom he is under greater obligations.

John Stuart Mill[2]

Nothing existing can be called "bad" insofar as it exists, but only insofar as it lacks or needs something. Thus a human might be called bad insofar as he lacks power or virtue, as an eye can be said to be "bad" insofar as it lacks the power of vision.

Thomas Aquinas[3]

INESCAPABLE PERSPECTIVES OF PERSONS

Ethics happens because there are persons in the world. Embodied in history and culture, a person's approach to ethics is necessarily shaped by context, cultural constructs, and psychological development. When we discuss or dispute ethical issues—whether in philosophy departments, in kitchens, or on the street—there is always more going on than a disagreement over evidence or facts. The discovery of this com-

plexity has been troubling enough to some thinkers that they have concluded that ethics has little or nothing to do with evidence or facts.
Schools of thought have been built on that conviction.

So have ways of life: "It's all a matter of taste." "Who's to say?"

So have political tactics: "It's an emotional issue." "It's ideological."

So have philosophers: For years, "emotivists" held sway in academic circles, insisting in one form or another that ethics was not a matter of factual evidence or cognitive investigation.

What I would reflect on, however, is not the theory of emotivism
or the appeal to relativism but something else. The inescapable reality is
that all of us approach the world we share from perspectives, by virtue
of the simple condition of being embodied in a particular space and
time. Moreover, each of us brings powerful dispositions about the
world. Although we may not be condemned to perspective and disposition, we certainly do not escape them. This is not bad. Nor is it particularly confined to ethics. It is the texture of everything persons do.

One of the common but hidden differences in the way people discuss ethical issues is that they are simply interested in different parts of
the situation. Their very approach is different, and their differing approaches, each with controlling interests or partial emphasis, subtly influence how they judge the rightness or wrongness of a particular action
and what they think is important to look at. Sometimes their interests
are so prevailing that they cannot even see data that someone else presents. Often they cannot comprehend another person's "point."

Each person brings an attitude, a feel, a sense of what matters or
what is most important in life, in work, and in one's choices. One could
likewise say that there are varying psychological dispositions that lead
different theoreticians to differing postures before they entertain any
philosophical or ethical questions. Are some of us psychologically inclined to a more analytic stance, to breaking down large issues into
manageable, even controllable parts? Do others of us incline to the syn-
thetic move, hungering for unity and wholeness? There is no doubt that
some thinkers are more at ease with order and structure, others more at
ease with contingency and diversity. The personality tests that identify
us as "sensers" and "judgers," "feelers" and "thinkers," are more than popular indicators of our dispositions. They also may suggest seemingly ir-
reconcilable starting points in ethics.[4]

The same questions have been raised with respect to gender. Carol
Gilligan has claimed that there is a "different voice" with which women

speak and address the world. Is the fact that some of us are more concerned with logic and principle, others of us more concerned with care and compassion, a function of gender?[5] One cannot deny the diversity of perspective, even if one does not think it is rooted in our sexual differences.

Personal dispositions—whether they are functions of gender, psychohistory, economic class, race, or power structure—surely influence how we organize our experience of the world and how we frame our questions about it. Yet we can bridge them if we can acknowledge them *as* perspectives and talk about them from the common ground of our solidarity as embodied, self-conscious beings.

The fact that there are different psychological, sociological, and economic factors that influence even the questions we ask is no scandal. It would be a scandal only if we thought that human persons or their minds were those "ahistorical" agents that so many ethicists seem to fear. What is universal and invariant is the fact that, regardless of the diversity of context, we have the commonly shared capacity to question, ethically or otherwise.

Diversity in the ways people approach ethical questions is exemplified perfectly in the history of ethics. One sees it most frequently in debates over the right and the good in morality. Often the contenders in an argument are simply interested in different things. They are sometimes set in hardened and untranslatable opposition to each other.

ACHIEVING THE MORAL GOOD AND DOING THE RIGHT THING

One of the more common polarities in culture, community, and classroom seems to be a conflict between pragmatic results and idealistic principles. On one hand are people who seem most interested in finding answers to questions about what choices will bring about the most good. This approach is expressed in questions concerning "the good life," or happiness and fulfillment, or the goal of our actions. Aims, goals, fulfillments, results—a cluster of teleological terms (*telos* meaning "end")—therefore have been associated with "teleological" ethics.

On the other hand are people who seem much more interested in finding out the *right* thing to do, no matter what the results may be. When issues of justice and rights cohere in the personal experience of "oughtness" or the motivation of duty (*deon*, in Greek), this approach frequently has been called "deontological."

To be sure, much more is going on in moral arguments and in ethical literature than the clash of opposing approaches to life. Moreover, the dichotomy sketched above does not adequately express the differences. A teleologist, for example, will point out that she is interested in the "right" thing to do but that she uses a "goals and results" principle to reach the right thing. A deontologist could say that he is concerned with the internal requirements of duty but that these requirements indicate what is truly good.

Be that as it may, there is a strong difference in orientation and approach, even in the more sophisticated debates about morality, and this orientation surely is influential in our everyday political discussions and ethical debates. More concretely, the opposing stances or approaches to ethics could be formulated this way: What is fulfilling and what will make me (or us) happy is one question. What should I do, what ought I do, what is the right thing is another. In other words: *Telos* says, "The *good* is what is right to do." *Deon* says, "What I *ought* to do will be morally good."

In classrooms, on talk shows, in sophisticated articles, and on op-ed pages, one can feel the pull in two directions:

- What will make me happy? What is the best for all of us? What will bring about the greatest good for all involved?
- What are your (my partner, my company, my tribe, my nation) duties? This approach—at least today—is taken less rarely with respect to *my* duties. This particular gap in the application of duties and responsibilities, however, may be a function of our culture or something else.

As many readers will recognize, the great classical examples of these approaches are Mill and Kant—two figures who dominate introductory texts in ethics as much as they haunt discussions and articles of most professional ethicists. Scholars of Mill and Kant also will recognize that my allusions to their two traditions are at best merely representative of a standard account that does full justice neither to the original thinkers nor to the developments within their traditions. I wish to reflect, however, on the divergence of emphasis and interest—especially when taken in an unnuanced way, or exemplified in culturally accepted opinion. The thinness of my treatment of Kant and Mill, then, is not so much a commentary on their work as it is an observation about how their approaches are expressed in the "received" wisdom of acculturated ethics. In this section, consequently, I offer not instruction but interpretation.

Mill's teleological ethics, focusing on the goal of happiness for the greatest number of people, marks much of the discussion concerning moral right and wrong. His libertarian concerns, as well, inhabit almost every ethical debate. Kant's emphasis on rationality and the experience of duty is less common, even rather strange today; his concern for the interior workings of moral consciousness and motivation are quite strongly with us, however—although not under the rule of reason or "oughtness." True, we hear from Spike Lee movies and presidential speeches that we must do the "right" thing, even though it may be hard, unpopular, or distasteful. *What* people think is the "right" thing, however, is rarely subjected to the rational rigor and honesty that Kant would require of us.

A third approach—not quite a duty-based or a happiness-based ethics—is that of Thomas Aquinas, whose tradition also is represented (at least underground) in a common legal and civic sensibility that appeals to intrinsic values. Men and women, on this account, are created equal, with inalienable rights that no "good" and no "duty" can override. Thus, Martin Luther King, Jr., would appeal to a higher law that trumps the so-called "good" of the community or the duties positive law might impose. Interestingly, in his "Letter from the Birmingham Jail," King cited not Kant or Mill but Aquinas.

These three thinkers and the traditions they embody are not set up as rigid opposing camps. In fact, their greatness derives from the fact that each strives to integrate the perspectives and claims of the other world-views. They do so, however, in their own ways. Thus, rather than engaging in the familiar tactic of contrasting arguments found in the ethical systems of Kant and Mill (and, to a much lesser extent, Aquinas), in this chapter I contrast three quite different *sensibilities* about ethical reality and its relation to the rest of the world.

Kant, Mill, and Aquinas—among other observations that one could make about them—have entirely different sensibilities about what is important and interesting. Their ethnicities alone—German, British, and Italian—are enough to channel their various entries into ethics. They may be looking *at* the same things, but they definitely are not looking *for* the same things. So it is with us all. The contrasting dispositions we bring to ethics, no matter how elegantly we rationalize them and no matter how sensibly we articulate them, usually haunt our ethical disputes.

We can easily find ourselves in hot argument over issues that seem so clear and yet are so muddled. As often as not, the muddling derives not from the facts at hand but the interest we bring to the facts. It influences our style, our debate, the evidence we are willing to entertain, the conclusions we are inclined to suggest. Right here, we run up against some of the strongest divergences in ethical discussion, whether that discussion relates to issues of care versus justice, immediacy versus rules, relationship versus norms, knowledge versus feeling, or internal factors versus external ones.

Kant and Mill can be taken to represent the two dominant psychological-ethical impulses that are the subtexts in most ethical debates. The traditions of both are strong, although in the United States (especially in our contemporary life), the teleological approach—of which Mill's utilitarianism was the most influential expression—seems to have achieved full ascendancy. The aspect of Kant that remains strong is not that of principle or ought or duty; it is the emphasis on *interior* aspects of the moral choice, especially *motivation*—the contemporary motivations most frequently approved being sincerity or "love" or freedom. This approach stresses our *internal* disposition, albeit not the one that Kant concentrated on: the disposition of duty.

This concern for the interior aspects of morality most dramatically contrasts Kant with Mill, who is so devoted to the *external* dimensions of moral choice. For Mill, as our early thematic chapter-citation points out, our interior dispositions have little to do with morality. What really count are the results or consequences for all involved—especially results that are beneficial to humanity. Beneficial results make an act morally good. Mill may be interested in the "right thing to do," but he turns outward to find out what it is. One could call these two approaches the pull to the internal and the push to the outside.

Complementary to these approaches, I propose to reconstruct a third approach or emphasis that has been taken in history. We might call this the "intrinsic" approach. This intrinsic approach holds that certain qualities about moral agents called persons are intrinsically important to ethical discussions, regardless of whether we "internally" feel or judge or think it to be so. Notions such as "good," "value," "worth," and "dignity" are not only functions of interior dispositions that humans may have (I "feel" good or worthy or dignified). Nor are they merely functions of usefulness (I am worthwhile because I am productive, performing, and effective). These notions are related to existence itself—and all the manifold expressions of existence. This approach also stresses that certain intentional acts, regardless of the external factors or the internal motives, are somehow profoundly evil in themselves—as much a moral lack to the human person as sight is to a person who cannot see.

I offer this third approach by suggesting the world-view and ethical "feel" of Thomas Aquinas, whose position does not eliminate the value of Mill's or Kant's so much as it complements them in a more capacious integration of the strengths of their theories as well as many others.

KANT AND THE PULL TO THE INTERIOR

Ultimately, Kant's emphasis on duty is an emphasis on motive. This emphasis makes sense. We know, whether we are trying to evaluate our own behavior or whether guilt is being established in a court room, that intent or motive is crucial in understanding the moral quality of our actions. Our personal dispositions, the interior state of mind, the subjective state of our intentions are intuitively significant to us. We easily confirm this intuition on further reflection. "I didn't know the gun was loaded" makes all the difference in some cases. Clearly if I didn't know the gun was loaded, I didn't mean to kill the victim. I could not intend the killing—and intent is preeminent in determining culpability.

There are all sorts of important interior motives for a moral act, however. The question is, What motive bestows the quality of goodness or rightness on my action?[6] Four of us may agree that motive is important; but we may have four different ideas about *what* motives are important when we act. One might think that anything is morally good, as long as it is done out of love. Another might think that sincerity is the crucial motivation in our acts. A third—especially in our contemporary emphasis on fulfillment—might think that personal happiness is the key to determining the moral value of a choice. Finally, one might hold that as long as you are doing what you *ought* to do, *because* you ought to do it, you are doing the moral thing (although this perspective is rare today).

Kant thought that only this last interior disposition or motive was central to morality. The particular motive he fixed on as foundational was the motive of doing the right thing, doing what we *ought* to do. Why should we do X? Because we experience the "should" of it. This is what Kant means when he says, "Nothing can possibly be conceived in the world, or even out of it, which can be called good without qualification, except a good Will." That good will is a will that wills what it ought.[7]

Kant had an abiding conviction (which, I am prepared to argue, was at least halfway right) that the one quality that was constitutive to and inhabited every moral choice was the quality of "oughtness." He was convinced, therefore, that the very *meaning and rationale*, the very *intelligibility* of morality was "oughtness." Whether we choose to do X for pleasure's sake, for country, for fulfillment, for service or benevolence, or for our own egos, the underlying issue, no matter what alternative we settle upon, is what ought we do. Hedonists, egoists, naturalists, theists, and atheists have one thing in common when they are looking into morality. They are looking into what they *ought* do.

Doing what one ought to do, because one ought to do it, makes an act morally good. Our interior disposition says it all. Without the experience of *ought*, morality and ethics would make no sense. For Kant, neither tradition, nor context, nor fulfillment, nor personal need or pleasure, nor human nature makes an act morally good. Only the right motive of doing what one knows one ought to do could qualify an action for moral goodness. The only "good" without qualification is a good will: a will directed toward the doing of one's duty.

The very experience of morality, the very experience of having a moral *ought*, moreover, provides content to what we ought to do.

Duty is first of all an experience of *universality*. It is the one quality that characterizes every moral choice and option. There is no exception to this experience: No matter what our ethical position, no matter what norms or values we appeal to, the issue of duty is what we are all encountering and trying to solve. To respond to duty is to respond to the universal nature of moral experience.

Kant's first law was the logical expression of the universality experienced in ethics: *Never act in a way that one's principle or maxim could not be made into a universal law.* This law may seem abstract, indeed; yet "universality" is one of the earliest insights that makes moral sense to us as children. Who has not heard, "All the kids do it"? Who has not heard the parental form of the argument: "What if everybody did what you're doing?"

Every experience of morality also is an experience of our moral agency, our status as moral actors capable of moral choice. The very moment of moral engagement is a moment when we exercise and affirm our dignity as moral agents. We cannot even make a moral choice without making an implicit affirmation of personal dignity. Kant's second formulation of the moral law, consequently, embodies the affirmation of personal dignity that any moral choice entails. Among the ways this second formulation could be expressed: *Never treat a person as if he or she were a mere nonperson,* or *always act with respect to moral agents in such a way that they are treated as ends-in-themselves.*

Kant's turn to the internal logic of moral choice is indeed an emphasis on the subject who acts. Yet because it is a logic of moral action, it is in no way "subjective" or relativist. In fact, it proposes the most rigorous of demands upon us—based on the objective conditions of moral consciousness and the requirement of universality, without which morality would not make sense.

The "subject" has center stage in Kant's moral arena—but only from the point of view of those invariant, objective, and universal conditions that make being a "subject" or moral actor possible. In all of this, however, an *internal* phenomenon—one's motive—as an interior disposition, determines the moral nature of an action. In Kant's case, the signal motive, the only authentic ethical intention, is duty.

As we shall see, this "internal turn" need not have the Kantian twist—or Kant's very sophisticated and rigorous correctives. Other interior motives—love, sincerity, self-indulgence—can be selected as foundational in ethics, although Kant judged that logically impossible.

Kant's enthronement of duty is just the opposite of any motive that might be highly relative to the individual. It relentlessly challenges our relative subjective states, our needs, our feelings, our hopes for fulfillment. In fact, the interior dispositions of sincerity or love or even compassion have little to do with the ethical quality of our actions. For Kant, if I, as a priest, remain faithful to my vows because I find the priesthood a fulfilling and happy way of life, my choice has no moral quality at all. If I remain faithful, however, despite my desires to the contrary, despite my lack of fulfillment and enjoyment in my life, that fidelity alone has moral quality. If this analysis seems strange, consider the following questions: When do you really know when you have a friend? When she is happy being around you? When he finds it fulfilling? Or is it in difficult times, when she or he stands by you and is faithful to the friendship?

For Kant (at least at first sight), feelings have nothing to do with moral reflection and behavior. The formal and universal requirements of ethical reason have everything to do with it. Moreover, for Kant this assertion is an objective claim, admitting of no exceptions.

In contrast, most contemporary expressions of "internal" turning in ethics lead, more frequently than not, to positions that are less rigorous and objectivist than Kant's. The most exasperating and vivid remembrance I have of such internal relativism is the phrase of a friend who deserted spouse and children: "I had to do it. I had a duty to myself. I was unhappy, and it was best for all of us." I saw an unassailable wall of privatized motive.

A common perspective tied my friend to Kant, however. Whether one focuses on duty or any other internal disposition, the arena in which the contest of moral action takes place is within the highly valorized interior world of the one who acts.

MILL AND THE PULL OUTWARD

In contrast to an internal focus is the emphasis on conditions that are external to the person acting. Tradition, situation, positive law, peer group, and a host of other circumstances pull our moral attention to sources outside the moral agent, outside our reason and desire, even outside (as Mill reminds us in another of this chapter's lead quotations) our motives. Regardless of whether you do something good for duty, money, or fame, it is good if certain conditions are met.

If one wishes to maintain that the good or bad of a moral act depends wholly on the external factor of context, one can choose among a variety of relative standards.[8] Usually the phrase "it all depends . . ." introduces the particular circumstance or circumstances that a person finds most important.

In many ways, traditionalist or customary moralities have this external emphasis, whether one thinks a thing is morally right because it has always been done that way or because "we" do it that way, or because the "powers that be" deem it so: In each case, we are focusing on a source that is external to the agent to determine whether an act is right or wrong.

Similarly, cultural relativism provides a strong emphasis on the externalities of moral action. Some of us might claim that any given cultural, class, religious, national, or ethnic "ethos" is what ethics is all about. Others might insist that the rules of the social game or commonly accepted rules for discourse provide the criteria of moral good and evil. The stronger and more exclusive the emphasis is on culturally relative beliefs, the stronger and more exclusive is the contextual and circumstantial emphasis in ethics.

Finally, the emphasis on external circumstantial factors can be pushed to its extreme. One can insist that each case is so utterly unique in surroundings and context that there are no objective or intersubjective norms, no standards or values that might challenge a particular position. In this case, one would not be claiming that internal, "subjective" factors entirely determine the moral life. Instead, one would be focusing exclusively on unique external determinants that relativize the moral quality of action.

Among the broad range of contextual or external factors that people have chosen as the key to moral quality and the focus for ethical discussion has been the *result* that a particular act brings about. On this view, the consequences of an action reveal its moral goodness or badness. Even here, there could be a vast spectrum of particular consequences, any one of which one could focus on as the central issue in ethics talk. Whatever produces love or pleasure or righteousness or fulfillment or even my own vanity might serve as the external factor that determines moral quality.

For Mill—who serves somewhat as the gravitational point for the external turn in morality—the particular consequence of happiness gives an act moral goodness.[9] Results, on the utilitarian account, are what ethics is all about. The particular resultant of maximal happiness was Mill's primary concern, even though his rendering of *happiness* involved a sophisticated and nuanced expansion of the meanings of pleasure and fulfillment. Mill simply stated that "the creed which accepts as the foundation of morals *utility*, or *the greatest happiness principle*, holds that actions are right in proportion as they tend to promote happiness, wrong as they tend to produce the reverse of happiness."[10]

Personal subjective intentions such as sincerity, love, or duty count for little. What counts are the consequences of an action. As Mill reminds us (in one of the quotations at the beginning of this chapter), saving someone is morally right, no matter what the motive—duty included. Of all the possible "external" candidates that might be considered centrally crucial to moral right or wrong, Mill and the utilitarians—as well as those who would call themselves "consequentialists"—give primacy to the end results, whether they are construed under the rubric of the greatest happiness or the greatest good for the greatest number of people.

Motives are not meaningless or totally inconsequential for Mill, however. The point is that he interprets them and approaches them through the prior moral grid of proportionally weighed good consequences. Indeed, this is the way he reaches out to incorporate those who criticize utilitarianism as a "creed for swine" (the resulting happiness for a human is radically other than the resulting happiness for pigs). This is the way he opens his thought to pious Christians ("Do unto others as you would have them do unto you" is a results- and happiness-based injunction). This is the way he entertains any refinement of utilitarian principle.

Just as Kant does not ignore but incorporates the interests of "externalists" into his internal grid, so Mill attempts to provide an approach that is large enough to include other positions and perspectives. Mill concentrates on the objective qualities of a moral act, not wanting to confuse them with subjective dispositions. Kant enlarges the interior (albeit rational) component of morality so broadly that it almost consumes any objective or outward interest.

In both cases, the openness to alternative approaches is conditioned on the requirement that the alternatives pass through the affective grid of "dutiful intentions" or "desirable results." The power of these traditions is grounded in their expanse and capaciousness: There is no moral act absent the experience of duty; there is no moral act that is not placed, in some way, for the purpose of bringing about a good result.

Although these observations are in no way meant to be a critical review or evaluation of Kant and Mill in their texts or scholarly traditions, a question at least remains in the context of ethical dispositions that orient our attention to either internal structures of moral consciousness or the external effects of our actions. Might either approach be too constraining if we want to attend to the full range of moral experience?

THE PERSONAL CENTER

Can the moral world of a human being really have little or nothing to do with our fulfillments? Is it possible that the joy of a man or woman who is pleased and gratified by fidelity is inconsequential to the moral life? Is the fact that someone finds virtue attractive or integrity appealing of dubious ethical value? If I cherish life and love being a good parent, is that utterly unimportant to the moral realm? Such an extreme reading of Kant is appalling not only to the follower of Mill. It is counterintuitive, to say the least. It certainly seems coldly inhuman.

At the same time, one need not be a Kantian to find the notion that the moral quality of saving a person from drowning has nothing to do with motive somewhat experientially strange. The idea that there is little moral difference in life-saving done out of duty, self-aggrandizement, money, or love of the person is an odd presumption, to say the least. The conclusion that the greatest good might be attained by violating either our most fundamental duties or the most basic rights of a human person is troubling, at least. Some of the stronger defenses of slavery in the United States and the use of the atomic bomb in the war against Japan have been grounded in greater good arguments. These very choices, however, remind us of our deepest moral wounds. Nor can we say that utilitarians have not addressed these problems; they have. The grid of external consequence is just too rigid, however, for the rich and thick density of moral behavior to be jammed through. We are thrown back to consider human motive—and human identity.

The constraints that each tradition puts upon us may well be little other than constraints on our humanity. Internal and external turns alike isolate and intensify one part of the personal world and call it ethics. Yet an action can only be "ethical" because of the existing human beings who generate the ethical impulse in the first place.

The experience of "ought" is indeed a universal component of ethical experience. This experience does not happen in a vacuum, however. It happens in an ethical experiencer. Indeed, Kant gives privileged place to the moral agent in a kingdom of ends—but only as derived from the laws of moral logic. Kant stands in need of an ethical "turning right side up": someone to play Marx to his Hegel. The only reason there is a moral world is this: There are agents who introduce morality to the world. Duty does not spin out the dignity of persons. Persons spin out the reality of duty.

There are contended issues here, admittedly. These issues are related to the heavy questions of metaphysics and ontology. We cannot let the presumption of metaphysical "impossibilities" prevent us, however, from admitting that the concrete, existential person of flesh and blood does ethics. Ethics does not do us.

As we have seen, we are not ahistorical beings possessed of some airy essence. We are embodied, self-conscious beings lodged in history. Among our endowments are Kant's reason, both pure and practical. We are the kinds of beings that have such capacities. These capacities enable us to ask ethical questions and do moral right or wrong.

Mill himself knew this. His whole effort to defend utilitarianism against those who claimed that his doctrine degraded us was based on a conviction that human beings are a special *kind of animal*, with different capacities, needs, and fulfillments. What differentiates a pig, whether satisfied or dissatisfied, from a human being is the fact that the pig is constituted differently than the human. How else can Mill or anyone else speak of "higher" faculties in men and women? Every tactic that Mill employs has a hidden appeal to the ontological reality of human existence—to the very structure of our humanness, uniquely realized in each of us, commonly shared by all of us.

The nub of the Utility Principle is this: What is happiness for human beings? Fulfillments, consummations, satisfactions are meaningless unless they are anchored in the kind of being one is hoping to make happy. In Mill, as in Kant, there is a great return required. It is a return to the intrinsic conditions of human personhood that make duty experienceable and happiness affirmable.

This is why we have found it necessary to articulate a phenomenology of the human person as the originator of ethics. Yet such a move is not intended to enthrone the individual human as the center of the world. It is to acknowledge the existential reality of personhood, which is actually independent of our personal projections or desires.

THE INTRINSIC TURN

What if values and goods, moral or otherwise, are not only functions of human intention? What if they involve more than the disposition of our wills or the range of our fulfillments? What if values and goods are also realities to be discovered, to be acknowledged and appreciated, regardless of our intent or their usefulness?

Among the other ethical dispositions that can be found in the history of philosophy—and even among personality types—is a human sensibility that sees and encounters the world as charged with value and goodness in itself. Another way of putting it would be to challenge our anthropocentric view of the world. Without humans, would the earth not have goodness? Are we the exclusive bestowers of value on animals and flora, or do they have value whether we recognize it or not? Does not the land and its living beings have its own truth? And even if you were to insist that there must be intelligence for there to be truth and there must be will for there to be goodness that is loved, must it only be a human kind of intellect and will to affirm the truth and goodness of the cosmos?

Interestingly, in the "postmodern" removal of the imperial human ego from center stage, there are still very few people, especially philosophers, who are willing to entertain the possibility that there is an intrinsic value and goodness to existence itself—and that this value is not dependent on human fiat or construction.

There are as many varieties of this "intrinsic" turn as there are varieties of the internal and external turns. There also are considerable metaphysical and epistemological issues lurking here, of course. This circumstance is no more daunting, however, than the questions of reality and knowledge that haunt the approaches of Mill and Kant. Therefore, rather than discuss the epistemological and ontological commitments of a particular ethicist or review a particular line of moral argument, I examine here the *approach* of one philosopher—Thomas Aquinas—who makes the intrinsic turn in ethics.

Even more than Kant and Mill, Aquinas' historical and cultural contexts are utterly different from our own. His ethical theory, moreover, is intimately related to a theological and anthropological view of the cosmos that is profoundly alien to postmodern sensibility and dogma. Like Kant and Mill, however, Aquinas represents an approach to reality and ethics that is instanced over a wide range of thinkers and ages.[11] His approach still can engage human consciousness.

For Aquinas, notions of "good" and "ought" are married to the notion of existence itself. It is good and appropriate that things be and that they be what they are. The "matchmaker" of this marriage, at least within the domain of experience, is the human agent. Humans make this connection because they are endowed with cognitive capacities to know the existing world, to judge it and name it in all its diversity and continuity. They also are endowed with affective and volitional capacities to affirm and desire this world as desirable, worthwhile, and good in itself. Humans can freely say *yes* to the intrinsic value of beings in the world.

I can look at a forest and see it in terms of particular choices I might make about it. I can see it, more concretely, in terms of its relation to human fulfillments ("Wow: Think of all the newsprint and toilet paper we can sell!" or "Just imagine how important this rainforest is for ecological balance"). I can also look at a forest and encounter it with my appreciative judgments, however, affirming its beauty as a value in itself. I can contemplate its good and simply say *yes* to it. I can self-consciously appreciate the goodness and value of existing things. I can love them.

Aquinas actually *grounds* our concerns for "global diversity." Long before that term was invented, he maintained that every existing thing is in some way good—worthy of being an object of desire (or being desired into existence), affirmable in its own unique giftedness (or what Aquinas might call "perfection," a being's own special completion in itself). A flourishing horse has the full intrinsic goodness and completion of being a horse, even though it is not all horses, even though it is not a pig, even though a human might not appreciate it.

Each existing thing has value and goodness not only by the fact of its gift of existence—the fact that it actually *is*—but also by the fact of its existing as a particular *kind* of being, gifted with its own form that it might share with others of its kind. Each is also uniquely gifted as a *particularly existing member of its kind.*

A palomino is affirmable, good in itself, valuable intrinsically. Its very existence is its primary good and value, for if it did not exist, it could not be good or valuable in any other analogous sense of those words. We could not choose it. We could not use it. Without the primal good of existence, it could have no other perfections or gifts, for existence is the gift of gifts, the good of goods, without which there would be no secondary gift or good at all.

The palomino also is affirmable or good as a horse. The kinds of beings called horses are irreplaceable perfections or gifts in existence. Without the kind we call "horses," the world would not only be a different world; it would also be existentially poorer, for want of horses. To be sure, the grand march of species is a living parade of contingent, non-necessary goods. Each of the myriad species lost, however, is an existential loss—at the very least, in terms of the species itself. The loss of a species, which itself may be a necessary component of any evolving, living world, is nonetheless a loss because of the intrinsic good of life, in all its forms. Ultimately, I believe that this is the strongest reason why many people have concern for even the least consequential endangered species.

Finally, the palomino named Ajax is good not only because he *exists*, not only because he is a *horse*, but because he is singly and irreplaceably *Ajax*, unique in space and time. All existence—even on the level of this one species and this particular horse—is charged with value. Existence, the horse kingdom, and this horse have intrinsic goodness. Each level of itself is a perfection, an existential gift in the world. If there were no horses, even if there were no Ajax, there would be an existential loss of goodness on the earth.

This philosophical "worldview" and interest (which actually is much more metaphysically sophisticated than my discussion suggests) inhabits Aquinas' pre-ethical and ontological encounter with the universe. Not only do I recommend it as an intrinsic theory of ontic value, I also propose it as an important dimension for a fully robust theory of ethical value.

One might object that if this way of looking at the world is sound, what does one make of evil in the world? How can one affirm that existence is primarily and radically good in the face of horrible natural disasters, terrible physical disfigurement, and monstrous behaviors of humans? Is evil not real? Are there not "bad" or "undesirable" or ungood things and happenings in the world? Obviously there are, but every evil is known as such only in comparison to some experience of goodness. In fact, something is bad only insofar as it lacks goodness. Only insofar as it lacks existence in some way. Only insofar as it is deprived of its full perfection. Only insofar as there is something about it that is not desirable or affirmable.

Evil, whether physical or moral, is always in some way a lack in being, a hole in existence, a negation. In other words, it is essentially parasitic because it cannot exist except in a being that has the goodness of existence. Although not all lacks or limits are evil, every evil is a lack and privation. Thus, a man might be personally evil by his lack of an appropriate virtue or experience physical evil because of a lack in one of his organic powers.

An intuitive wisdom is present when we say "I have bad eyes." Aquinas calls visual deficiency a physical "evil," with no moral overtones whatsoever. Nor is such evil always a big deal. A spectrum of "badness" could be applied to my eyes, from slight nearsightedness to full blindness. In every case, however, we are speaking of a lack or deprivation. It is quite real. Its entire reality, however, is based on the perfection, the existence, of functioning eyes that partially enable the experience of sight.[12] In a way, we confirm this way of thinking with the use of words such as *disfunction* or *misuse.* The "dis" and "mis" are simple indicators of lack or privation.

The goodness and perfection of the function is always in relation to the appropriate state of the being in question. Some of our "lacks" actually are the good of being limited beings. They are not the lack of anything proper to us as the kind of beings we are. Not all lacks are evil, but all evils are lacks. An acorn may lack the fullness of all existing perfection; it may even lack the full good of the oak. As acorn, however, it has its own appropriate existential goodness and function (which neither humans nor oak trees have.)[13]

Persons, then, like all existing things, have intrinsic value and ontological goodness: the intrinsic value and goodness of existence, of being human, and of being individually embodied, reflectively conscious careers. Because human endowments capacitate them to introduce ethics into the world, however, in addition to the analogous goodness they share with all species there is an intrinsic moral quality about human lives and an ethical dimension to their desires and interests.

Consequently, everything that exists is affirmable. Each diverse existent has its own proper goodness. In Aquinas's view, the affirmation of the truth of a being, the affirmation of its own goodness, is what love is all about. In fact, for Aquinas, for something to even exist it must be loved into existence. Moreover, the tendency of each thing to maintain itself in existence is its own proper love of its existential reality. (Dante, in the *Paradiso*, called it the love that moves the stars and the human heart. Darwin might have called such "love" the hidden logic of the universal tendency for self-maintenance and survival.)

So far, however, this "intrinsic" turn to goodness is concerned with existence. The issue of moral good and evil emerges only in the realm of human *action.* The class of beings called "human" introduces, at least to the extent of our knowledge, moral, good, and evil into the world. Existential evil, as we have seen, is a lack, a privation of the goodness of existence. One could call this physical evil. A lack, a privation, a negation of being that is *consciously* and *freely* chosen is more than a physical evil, however. It is moral evil.

It is a physical evil that a horse be lame. It could well be a moral evil if a free agent chose to make the horse lame. It is a physical evil that organisms die (although it might be a good in a broader context of eco-system relationships). The question of moral evil occurs when the death is a result of free choice. As opposed to other kinds of beings that have no other choice but to be what they are, humans are a kind of beings that need not be what they are. Endowed with the capacity for self-understanding and self-definition, humans may consciously reject, deny, or negate what they are.

Humans are a special kind of being, bringing their own natural diversity to the world. Like other kinds of beings, they have a shared nature—but it is a free nature. Humans have a moral nature, a personal nature. They are not forced to be true to themselves. They are the kind of beings who are capable of self-consciously possessing their own life-story, of being not only biographies, but of embodying autobiography. The endowments of personal animals are not only existentially good. The privations of our lives are not only ontological or physical. They also have moral weight. We humans introduce moral goodness into the world. We also introduce moral lack, moral privation: moral evil.

This moral dimension characterizes the intrinsic value of persons as endowed moral animals in the world. The experience of "ought" occurs because of our constitution as personal natures, moral natures. "Ought" is experienced only by beings that do not automatically act out the truth of what they are. The questions of ethics can be raised only by the kinds of beings who are capacitated to question themselves and their world.

Motives are important to the moral world and to ethical discourse because persons are motive-bearing natures. We can have reasons and intentions for doing the things we do. Insofar as these motives touch on the truth and affirmation of our personhood, they have ethical weight. Kant was correct—certainly to the extent that the universal experience of "ought" is a universal experience of our personhood. *Consequences*, as well, are strategic to the moral world and to ethical discourse because our freely chosen actions have an impact on the existence of other persons and other beings in this world. The human person is inescapably situated in history and context and inevitably driven to seek fulfillment and flourishing, just as any natural being is. The consequence of happiness, moreover, is crucial—but only insofar as *humans* raise the issue and *humans* must discover what is truly beneficial for themselves, as the kinds of beings they are, and for other kinds of beings in the world.

The intrinsic turn in ethics does not negate the internal and external factors on which Kant and Mill focus. It seeks only to integrate them in a more capacious model of ethical discourse and behavior that is grounded in personal nature. We human persons—embodied, self-conscious beings—must have the same vigilance over our interior world that Kant had. We also must be as vigilant as Mill in the external turn to society, history, and culture. For our very nature is to bridge the internal and external worlds—not as ahistorical natures but as embodied beings.[14]

KILLING, AUTONOMY, AND INTRINSIC VALUES

In this section, I apply what I have been discussing to a case of intentional killing of persons. To clarify the discussion, I first distinguish what I mean by killing, intentional killing, and the murder of a person.

A *killing* can occur without any intent. A landslide may kill. A tiger may kill as well. (If you believe that tigers have the intent to kill, it must not be in the sense that "intent" requires knowledge of what one is doing and self-conscious ownership or responsibility for behavior—unless you think that tigers are capable of morally culpable acts.) Humans also kill unintentionally, or premorally, as in an accidental overdose or an accidental automobile crash—although there may be morally germane intents other than killing involved. This kind of killing is "premoral" in the true meaning of the word.

Intentional killing, as I use the term, means that you know you are killing a person, and you freely choose to do so. A moral act cannot even be placed without "informed consent," entailing knowledge and responsibility. Most people find this kind of killing justifiable at times, whether the killing is done for some required motive or for some desired maximal good. Intent, on this reading, is not the same as motive. One may intend to kill a person out of love or out of jealousy. The intent is the same; the motive, often mitigating, is different. I reject the intent to kill persons as a morally good act under any motive or consequence.

I generally do not use the term *murder* because it is intimately tied up with legal definitions and procedures. For example, murder may require malicious hatred as a motive. I believe that a person may choose the unethical killing of someone and yet have a noble motive or exalted cause. This act would not be murder, then—though I still argue that it is a profound violation of the moral order.

Although I have stressed the complementarity of ethical approaches, I believe an example of intentional killing significantly distinguishes the "intrinsic" approach from the other two. As a sample contrast, I offer the case of Timothy McVeigh and the Oklahoma City bombing. Imagine McVeigh as a terrible or perfect Kantian or as a perfect or terrible utilitarian. Imagine, also, a third position: that the killing of innocent persons is intrinsically wrong, no matter how high or compelling one's sense of duty and no matter how beneficial the results.

An essay attributed to McVeigh appeared in *Media Bypass Magazine*. In that essay, this decorated U.S. Army veteran of the Persian Gulf War decries the hypocrisy of the United States for stockpiling "weapons of mass destruction"—and actually using them on Hiroshima and Naga-saki—while criticizing Saddam Hussein for having his own weapons. McVeigh then compares the bombing of Iraq and the killing of inno-cent children:

> Actually, there is a difference here. The administration has admitted to knowledge of the presence of children in or near Iraqi government buildings, yet they still proceed with their plans to bomb—saying they cannot be held responsible if children die. . . . Who are the true barbarians? In this instance, the people of the nation approve of bombing government employees because they are "guilty by association"—they are Iraqi government employees. In regard to the bombing in Oklahoma City, however, such logic is condemned.
>
> What motivates these seemingly contradictory positions? Do people think that government workers in Iraq are any less human than those in Oklahoma City? In this context, do people come to believe that the killing of foreigners is somehow different than the killing of Americans? . . .
>
> Unfortunately, the morality of killing is not so superficial. The truth is, the use of a truck, a plane, or a missile for the delivery of a weapon of mass destruction does not alter the nature of the act itself.[15]

Clearly, McVeigh is working toward an equal justification for the killing of innocent government workers or children, whether by truck or plane. The "nature of the act itself" is rendered acceptable (as he writes later in the essay) "as a means to an end," whether employed by American terror or anti-American terror; thus, McVeigh seems to be arguing in terms of the greatest good achieved. Whether McVeigh is a terrible utilitarian thinker or an astute one (for surely there are utilitarian arguments against the killing of innocents), he mounts his defense of killing in the name of greater goods—some of which, to McVeigh, are as considerable as the future of the country and the world.

Even if McVeigh were a Kantian (albeit a confused one), he might still be conflicted. For although he would seem to be reducing persons to the status of mere means, he might still argue that his maxim (or moral choice) could be rendered a universal law: As a last resort, to defend humanity, the killing of innocents ought to be permitted.

We do know this, however: If McVeigh operated from the ethical position that intentionally killing an innocent human person is intrinsically wrong, that it can never be justified by any motive or any consequence, then he could find no moral justification for his act. (This assertion also would apply to U.S. government decisions to "terror bomb" Europe and Japan during World War II or to wage a "Desert Storm" against Iraq.) The point here is not that the third alternative is, in fact, the correct one. (I argue that later.) The point is that McVeigh cannot possibly use the third alternative alone to justify his actions.

Such an observation serves neither to defend McVeigh nor to impugn Kantianism or consequentialism. It simply points out that although internal or external emphases on ethical standards might justify the bombing in Oklahoma or Baghdad, a theory of intrinsic right and wrong could not.

Another contrasting example of the three approaches is in the area of "autonomy." Because *autonomy* is a concept used by Kant in a manner that is logically related to the very experience of moral consciousness, it is subject, on his account, to the constraints of categorical imperatives. Kant does not ground the notion in the endowed constitution of human nature, however; now that "autonomy" is set free from the restraints of Kant's moral logic, it survives culturally as an honorific term. Although "autonomy" is relatively common in political discourse and medical ethics discussion of informed consent, the related concept of "liberty" is far more dominant in contemporary moral consciousness. This is clearly more Mill's contribution.

In the introduction to *On Liberty*, Mill states simply: "In the part [of conduct] which merely concerns himself, his independence is, of right, absolute. Over himself, over his own body and mind, the individual is sovereign." To be sure, Mill placed restraints on such sovereignty. It did not apply to children because of their immature faculties. It did not apply to "backward societies" or "barbarians." (This position is disconcerting from the great libertarian: an indication of culturally preferred sanctions on *certain* people's autonomy.)[16] Today, however, the "liberty principle" reigns with respect to matters of "one's own body and mind." In fact, many Supreme Court cases regarding the termination of fetal life and the choice of suicide involve direct appeals to the "liberty interest" of the individual.

The point to be made here, however, is that an intrinsic theory of right and wrong might well place constraints on one's autonomy, even with matters that concern one's own body. If one holds that killing oneself is intrinsically immoral, regardless of the intent or the positive outcome, suicide would be ethically impermissible.

For Aquinas, the moral universe is grounded in the intrinsic constitution of human persons. The kind of beings they are is a moral kind: a kind capable of self-consciously defining acts. Moreover, Aquinas sees the world—and especially persons—as intrinsically charged with premoral value and goodness. The world has value not by reason of our attribution but by reason of our recognition of its intrinsic goodness. Our free and deliberate encounter of this existentially good world sets the stage for morally good or evil action. Finally, in the context of moral choice, premoral intrinsic value and goodness—especially as found in the life of a human person—puts moral constraints on our actions and autonomy.

Moral action exhibits all of the characteristics that mark human persons as embodied, self-conscious beings in history. Moral action, as well as all moral discourse, must be capacious and integrated enough to mirror the fact that persons are subject to all the contingencies of space and time—and are critically and self-consciously aware of that fact. Persons can recognize and respond to the intrinsic value of existing diversity. They also are invariably motive-driven. Persons have intrinsic natural drives to fulfillment. Their moral task, in some ways like Kant's and Mill's, is to discover *what* motives, *what* fulfillments, are true to their personhood and true to the existential value of the human and nonhuman world around them. Failure in such a task is a moral failure. It is moral evil. Yet we remember that moral evil, like physical evil, never exists in itself. Evil has existence only in a borrowed way—only by inhabiting an ontologically good being.

Thus, evil is a parasite, and malice is essentially an emptiness, a negation. For Aquinas, therefore, love is absolutely more enduring than hate, good absolutely more permanent than evil.

Moral evil can enter the world only because there are existentially good beings, moral beings, human beings who are able to take their lives into their own hands through the endowments of intellect and will and choose to be true to their identity or not.

Humans can negate their truth. They can choose their own deprivation. They can embrace not the truth of their existence but a lie.

6
Before Good and Evil

The place of what I call skepticism in our culture is evident. By this I do not mean just a disbelief in morality, or a global challenge to its claims—though the seriousness with which a thinker like Nietzsche is regarded shows that this is no marginal position. I am also thinking of the widespread belief that moral positions cannot be argued, that moral differences cannot be arbitrated by reason, that when it comes to moral values, we all just ultimately have to plump for the ones which feel/seem best to us. . . . Ask any undergraduate class of beginners in philosophy, and the majority will claim to adhere to some form of subjectivism. This may not correspond to deeply felt convictions. It does seem to reflect, however, what these students regard as the intellectually respectable option.

Charles Taylor[1]

In the late 80s, while American academics were emptily theorizing that language and the thinking subject were dead, the longing for freedom and humanistic culture was demolishing the very pillars of European tyranny. Of course, if the Chinese students had read their Foucault they would have known that repression is inscribed in all language, their own included, and so they could have saved themselves the trouble of facing the tanks in Tiananmen Square. But did Vaclav Havel and his fellow playwrights free Czechoslovakia by quoting Derrida or Lyotard on the inscrutability of texts? Assuredly not: They did it by placing their faith in the transforming power of thought—by putting their shoulders to the immense wheel of the word. The world changes more deeply, widely, thrillingly than at any moment since 1917, perhaps since 1848, and The American Academic left keeps fretting about how phallocentricity is inscribed in Dickens's portrayal of Little Nell.

Robert Hughes[2]

The world today is a world in which generality, objectivity and universality are in crisis. . . . And when a personal tone does crop up, it is usually calculated, not an outburst of personal authenticity.

Sooner or later politics will be faced with the task of finding a new, postmodern face. A politician must become a person again, someone who trusts not only a scientific representation and analysis of the world, but also the world itself. He must believe not only in sociological statistics but also in real people. He must trust not only an objective interpretation of reality, but also his own soul; not only an adopted ideology, but also his own thoughts; not only the summary reports he receives each morning, but also his own feeling.

Soul, individual spirituality, first-hand personal insight into things; the courage to be himself and go the way his conscience points, humility in the face of the mysterious order of Being, confidence in its natural direction and, above all, trust in his own subjectivity as his principal link with the subjectivity of the world—these are the qualities that politicians of the future should cultivate.

Vaclav Havel[3]

THE FIELD OF MORAL EXPERIENCE

The emphasis on the primacy of the personal subject in ethics can appear to be a form of the subjectivism that seems to reign from classrooms to the streets. "Who's to say what is right or wrong?" "No one can tell anyone else what he or she can or cannot do." "It's all a matter of feeling and perspective." "It's a personal matter." "You can't judge others." The relativism and skepticism that Charles Taylor describes, however, is not only in the minds of university undergraduates. As social critic Robert Hughes points out, it is an underlying presupposition in the trendiest seminars and the most bizarre talk shows. One might falsely presume that the emphasis on the "person" that characterizes this book would underwrite the relativism and subjectivism that Taylor and Hughes find in contemporary culture. The goal of this chapter is to show how that is not the case. A robust and thick theory of the human person, endowed with rational and affective capacities, yields a theory of human judgment that is open to the truth of the subject as well as the external world. Moreover, ethics will be seen not so much as a matter of the constructions we impose upon the world and our choices as an honest humility before the truth of our personhood, embodied in the world.

In this context, I examine the dynamics of moral judgment and moral failure as functions of our openness to the truth of what we are.

An emphasis on the human subject does not require a commitment to subjectivism or relativism, especially if one's notion of the human person is an integrated unity of body and reflexive consciousness. By this proposition, human persons are understood as neither isolated egos nor material objects. Their ethical world cannot be reduced to mere interior dispositions, functional utility, or external measurement. The personal world is a fusion of interior and exterior realities.

As embodied, we inhabit history and environments; we exist and develop by means of culture and interpersonal relations. There is no way for us to live and thrive as persons or selves other than as related to and dependent on a reality that is "other" than us, our perspectives, our wants. Thus, Vaclav Havel reminds us that a rejection of objectivity and universality is no guarantee of personal authenticity. The authentic person—the one who has passed through the perils of postmodern disillusionment not with despair but with humility—must have a trust in the world and objective interpretations of reality, as well as one's soul, mind, and feelings. Authentic subjectivity requires a faithfulness to the objective conditions of personhood and the world it inhabits.

This radical openness to the world of our interior endowments as well as the conditions of the world around is nothing other than the arena of conscience and the field of our moral experience.

In this chapter, then, I examine the field of moral experience and how its constituents permeate each other in that moment of moral judgment called "conscience." Moral experience itself provides a fundamental standard as close to us as fidelity to and love of the truth of who and what we are. Finally, I consider, through the works of two artists, the price we pay for rejecting and repressing our moral truth.

Any mapping of a personalist ethics must include the full range of our humanness as embodied, self-conscious beings. As self-conscious, our experience is inescapably subjective and internal. As embodied, however, our moral experience has external factors: the physicality of the body itself, the objective conditions of space and time, the intersubjective conditions of culture and context. Of course, these realms are not isolated from each other—or mutually opposed. They actually interpenetrate each other in the unified integrated personal being called an "embodied self-consciousness." For there is an "objectivity" to being a subject. There are intrinsic conditions required for self-consciousness,

interior feelings and judgments and intended action, whether I subjectively recognize them or not. The "external" world itself, of which I am
a part and which is a part of me, has its subjective conditions—in the
experience of subjects other than myself or in the symbolic forms of society or culture.[4]

Particular moral actions, then, take place in a dynamic relationship
of internal actions and dispositions and external contexts and influences. If I am considering the moral goodness or rightness of terminating a human's life, clearly I am doing the considering and I will make the
judgment. Motives and intentions that belong to me will be crucial. Just
as clearly, however, there are external factors that significantly modify
my action and judgment. For example, do I have any information? Who
is the person I am about to kill? What does my society teach and reward
with respect to killing? Is it really a person I am about to kill? What effects will this action have on me, my people, my society? Are there deficiencies in my judgment because of trauma to my own cognitive or affective system? Am I brainwashed or in a drug-induced stupor?

Issues with which Kantians and utilitarians concern themselves are
involved in all of these questions about the dynamic complexity of
moral action. Yet *all* of these questions are significant. No single particular context, result, motive, or internal or external factor exhausts or
completely covers the full moral quality of a human action. A moral
action is as complex as the human person who places it. So is the concrete moral judgment concerning "What ought I do?" in any particular
situation.

THE DYNAMICS OF PERSONAL MORAL JUDGMENT

Because human beings have a capacity for self-conscious, embodied activities, they are capable of intelligent affirmations and rational
judgments. Persons can bestow a freely given "yes" or "no" on themselves and the world. Thus, every affirmation, every consciously known
and possessed affirmative judgment, is open to a moral dimension,
wherein persons reveal a free response to their position in the world and
their relationships to each other.

Our judgments, actions, and affirmations are not mindless repeti-
tions of information or input. They are not merely mirrors of the culture
or society or family that formed us. What morally charges these actions

and judgments is that they reveal the stance, attitude, and free responsiveness of a human agent. A person owns his or her experience, judgments and actions. He or she is accountable for them.

Because these judgments are not forced or necessitated, they take the form of "I ought" or "I should." These judgments do not declare a mere state of affairs; they reveal a state of personally owned disposition. They are affirmations that are attributable only to the one who affirms. They are judgments of conscience: practical judgments of the form, "I ought to do this action."

This notion of conscience, consequently, is unlike that in Freud's *Civilization and Its Discontents*. Freud portrays conscience as something of an internal faculty—the product of introjected cultural and familial forces, always related to guilt and the negation of impulse.[5] The notion of conscience I offer here is more akin to that of Aquinas, who insists that conscience is not a "faculty" but the activity of judging. "Through our conscience we judge that something ought to be done or ought not to be done."[6] Conscience is grounded in human rationality and ought to be followed, even if it is based on misinformed judgment—although we surely should inform our judgments as best we can.

Indeed, the contents or data on which the judgment of conscience are made are to a great extent supplied by civilizing forces—but the capacity for moral judgment itself is not. Thus, conscience is not the voice of some tyrannical super-ego; it is the self-conscious judgment of Freud's "ego" or "intelligence," in which Freud himself places so much faith.

A judgment of conscience can be made only by the person who owns and utters it. It is of the person. Its reality depends on and derives only from the person who offers it. It is a preeminently personal judgment. No one can claim ownership of another's conscience. No book offers formulations of it. No "third agent" or Jimminy Cricket tells me what to do. No state or church can claim dominion over it; only by the free affirmation of one's willingness to attend to the doctrine of state or church can either make a claim on conscience.

I cannot really say "the Bible is my conscience," or "the civil law is my conscience," or "God's will is my conscience." I can only say that my own moral judgment is my conscience; I am the one who forms my judgment according to the Bible, the state, or the will of God. Only I, the human person, can affirm what I so affirm.

I don't do this in a vacuum, however. Whenever I exercise conscience or affirm moral judgment, I do so in the context of my historically embodied actuality and the content of my life-career. Like any other judgment, the judgment of conscience is highly dependent on the information I have received or pursued. It also is strategically modified by the misinformation that might be forced on me. All information is formation—not only of the embodied person but of the embodied person's further embodiments in moral action. Thus, in the formation of my moral judgment, my openness to data, to evidence, and to argument is as important as it would be in the formation of a legal judgment or a scientific judgment. Just as we would not trust the "business judgment" of someone who can give no rational account or evidence for a judgment made, just as we would expect the articulation of theory and application to data in scientific judgment, so also in moral judgment: "Judgment" itself is not enough. It must be warranted and grounded. If it is not, it is moral foolishness—if not bankruptcy.

Moral judgments, therefore, can be misinformed. They can be formed by distortions, lies, incomplete information, ignorance, or propaganda. Like any judgment, they can be distorted by fear, force, terror, deprivation, addiction, or psychological distress. Even in these cases, however, they are mine. As an individual agent, I can ultimately own and execute in action only my own judgment. And I can embody in moral behavior only my own conscience, misinformed or not. All such behaviors are revelations of my personal responsibility before the world; as such, they are moral.

Even if my moral judgments are perverse or malformed, they are preeminent in my moral life, for the only final indication of my moral quality as a person is the judgment I make concerning what ought to be done—and my personal fidelity to that judgment in my choices.

Indeed, it is central to ethics that one follow one's judgment. Just as central, however, is the requirement that one's moral judgment, one's conscience, not be that of a fool.[7]

THE SUBJECTIVE INTERNAL DIMENSION

If I have before me an action that I take as my own—an action that reveals my stance before others and the world and for which I am responsible—the only basis on which I can take action is my own judgment about its rightness or goodness. This is the preeminence of conscience.

Conscience is a primary expression of human freedom. It is rooted in the fact that we are the kind of beings endowed with special capacities of knowledge and freedom that charge our actions with moral quality.

Behind all appeals to "freedom of conscience" in all the diverse examples that we encounter across times and cultures and in all the pluralisms of class, race, or gender is the objective and universal reality of what being a human person means in the first place. "Freedom of conscience" is given such high privilege and "freedom of worship"—itself based on conscience—is so highly valued in the name of human personhood. We each ought to follow our own conscience in the name of human personhood, for our own moral judgment is the only moral judgment we have. To give up our conscience is to give up our moral judgment itself. It is to give up our moral freedom. It is to give up the ethical life. It is to reject personal life.

Because conscience is a preeminently personal activity, however, fully judging the moral life of other human beings is impossible. We may question their judgments. We may challenge the way they have formed their judgments. We cannot fully evaluate their moral character, however. Only if we know their own particular moral judgment or conscience—"I ought not cheat"—and we know they freely choose to do it anyway can we know that they are personally unethical in that action.

Moreover, the internal side of moral judgment includes a spectrum of possible motives and intentions that modify the quality of a moral act. A man may be a prostitute for the sake of love or money. Although the motive is not the whole story, it is part of it. A woman may be a killer for vanity or for justice's sake. Again, her motive may not be everything, but it does count for something.

Finally, internal conditions may profoundly affect the quality of a moral choice itself. My internal confusion or fear may seriously distort my judgment. Torture or threat radically modify my freedom. Physical trauma or lack of cognitive skills diminish my culpability. My culture, gender, and class all have bearing on my "own" internal moral judgment of conscience. Even normal psychological development affects the way I process information about the world and respond to it.[8]

"I didn't know the gun was loaded" is not merely a potential legal defense. It is an internal condition of ignorance that fundamentally alters the moral quality of an action. Premeditation and deliberateness are required for full culpability.

Thus, even in this privileged internal and "subjective" realm of human conscience, conscience cannot be what it is if it is not related to the so-called external and objective world of one's own body structure and environment, one's cultural and political systems, and, especially, the information one has received to provide the data for the judgments one makes.[9]

A truly "personal" moral act must turn to the external world of consequences, context, and evidence as well as the internal world of motive and intent.

THE OBJECTIVE EXTERNAL DIMENSION

Every human judgment is based on information—including our judgments about whether an act is morally good or right. Thus, conscience, however "subjective" it may be, is always based on information. Moreover, because we can be misinformed, our consciences (our ethical judgments), though subjectively assured they are certain, quite simply can be incorrect.

It is one thing to be sure you are morally right, to be certain that your conscience is true in your judging that, for example, apartheid is morally good. It is quite another to be correct. A sincere and sure racist has sincerity and surety—but that is not quite enough. There may be morally culpable and inculpable racists, depending on their knowledge of what they are actually involved in, their malice or lack of it, their circumstances and motives. Both, however, are involved in an objectively evil pattern of life that is not only challengeable but *must* be challenged. Similarly, there may be subjectively noble and ignoble killers, but both are acting in an objectively immoral way.

Noncognitivists or emotivists in ethics may insist that morality is solely a matter of emotion, feeling, or inclination, but that position, if tenable at all, can apply only to the level of first principles or the question whether we should be moral at all. Indeed, no one can be "argued" or "proved" into being morally upright. Logic and facts, by themselves, cannot deliver moral sensibility or choice.[10]

Logic and facts are crucial, however, to the very formation of the personal moral judgment itself. "Objectivity"—all of the dimensions of experience that are not reducible to my own needs, projections, and perspectives, the world of other persons, and nature itself—is as central to ethics as it is to any other human activity.

Objectivity does not mean agreement or universal acceptance of a state of affairs. Such "objectivity" is found neither in ethics nor in science or literature.[11] *Objectivity* does not necessarily mean that humans will think or judge the same way, but it does mean that humans are constituted the same way. It means that we can discover how we are constituted and endowed, even though these endowments are expressed in splendid variety. It means that there are facts about my human reality— whether I like it or not, whether I accept it or not, whether I know it or not.

No matter what my projections or preferences or feelings or motives about smoking, the fact is that smoking does something to my body. The Philip Morris Company may have spent years and millions of dollars to deny this fact, but their denial did not alter the reality. It was an objective reality before we ever knew the data. Now that I know the data, it is important in the formation of my moral judgment about whether I ought to continue smoking. If I resist or repress this evidence, I am betraying the proper function of moral judgment itself.

Objectivity does not mean that a given moral position somehow forces agreement or convinces. Every human utterance is assailable, limited, and deniable. Not every human utterance, however, is wholly relative, subjective, emotive, or reducible to cultural conditioning.

To claim objectivity as part of ethics is to claim that evidence about the world, the ozone layer, the development of the fetus, the behavior of animals, or the function of carcinogens is significant in the formation of moral judgments concerning ecological responsibility, animal "rights," and unhealthy behaviors. It is to claim that there are data about what it means to be a person, about the functioning of the human body, about the dynamics of human sexuality, and especially about the conditions required to have a conscience or freedom in the first place.[12]

One can also claim "objectively" that the value or worth of a human person is not a function of subjective preference, color, attractiveness, state benediction, productivity, personal sentiment, or economic standing but is an intrinsic property. Humans, by the very fact of being human, are endowed with the intrinsic value of personhood.

To claim objectivity as part of ethics is to claim that the information we receive from our culture or our economic class is open to question and is challengeable by data that the culture or class has not considered or may not want to consider.

During a visit to South Africa, I had the opportunity to hear and visit with Beyers Naude—a prominent Afrikaner, member of the famous Bruderbund, and onetime leader of the Dutch Reformed Church. Named after one of the great generals from the Boer War, Naude might likely have risen to the head of his church or even his nation. In his middle years, however, he undertook a personal investigation of the Christian scriptures to determine whether apartheid—which he had been taught was "the will of God"—could be justified by an encounter with the evidence of the Gospels.

Naude discovered that there was no other way to evaluate apartheid than as a sin, a rejection of the teachings of Jesus. The evidence overwhelmed him. If he were to follow his conscience, to be faithful to his own moral judgment, he knew he would put his reputation, his profession, and even his family into jeopardy. His judgment of conscience was based not on what he preferred doing, not on what might bring happiness to him, his people, or even his nation, but on what the evidence led him to judge. Apartheid was not only a denial of the intrinsic dignity of the human person; it was a denial of the standards that Naude himself had guided his life by and the revelation of the God he worshipped.

When Naude announced his opposition to apartheid, he was ejected from the white Dutch Reformed Church, removed from the Afrikaner leadership, and eventually "banned" within his own homeland. His professional sacrifice was offered not at the shrine of expediency, not at the altar of a universalizable proposition, but in the name of intrinsic human rights and the religious commitment that grounded those rights. The evidence demanded it.[13]

Evidence is critical in arriving at judgment. Moreover, if one is open to it, evidence can challenge and change one's conscience.

In a lecture on Christian foundations for nonviolence, I proposed to a group of believers that if one seriously wanted to follow the way of Christ, one might be drawn eventually to a position opposing capital punishment. In the discussion that followed, an older woman from the back of the audience challenged my position as "liberal" rather than Christian, saying, "After all, even Jesus said, 'an eye for an eye, a tooth for a tooth.'"

This woman was basing her "conscience" on that evidence. Although she may well have been certain in her convictions, her conscience, her judgment, was incorrectly informed. In fact, because she was willing to look at the actual evidence to which she was appealing, she found in Matthew 5:38 that Jesus was saying just the opposite of what she had been led to believe.

This new information did not solve the moral issue automatically, of course. The woman would look for further evidence. She also would reexamine her principles: Perhaps she would prefer to follow Leviticus instead of the gospel of Matthew. If her foundational principle would remain that she would follow the way of Jesus, she would have to change her conscience. That she did.

The foregoing examples highlight the strong cognitive and evidential contributions to personal conscience. They also reveal how strongly an "individual" and private phenomenon such as conscience (as well as our "selves") is informed by our relationships and our social world. Although moral judgments are made possible by the intrinsic endowments of personhood, they are never spun out of some interior citadel called the self. We cannot even *be* a "self" without others and without the cultural systems of meaning we build.[14]

CONTEXT, CULTURE, AND PERSONAL CHALLENGE

Entire cultures and traditions can be wrong. They can be wrong in the sense of being misinformed or incorrect with respect to the information they are built on. They also can be morally wrong with regard to the corporate behavioral practices that are based on the misinformation. Moreover, the moral flaw of a culture is compounded if the misinformation of its people—its disinformation—is corporately orchestrated to repress the truth, as in the Third Reich, Stalin's Russia, and Pol Pot's Cambodia. It happens in our own nation as well—whenever, because of cultural propaganda, we are willing to render the human person expendable in the name of our own self-interest.

Cultures and traditions, to be sure, nurture us in the formation of our very identity, our sense of who we are, and our convictions about right and wrong. We would have no content about anything if we were not cultivated by others and sustained by the linguistic, symbolic, and narrative information our society gives us. Our culture, however, does not give us our human personhood with its intrinsic endowments, through which culture itself has come into existence. Culture is the *ex-*

pression of embodied, self-conscious beings. Cultures and traditions are *built* by humans who, of course, were nurtured by culture. Every new personal entry into culture, every child born with personal endowments, is by its nature a challenge to any part of culture that represses or denies our human personhood.

Thus, when Gandhi professed that he would never sacrifice Truth even for the defense of his country, he was welcoming the challenge of conscience to the patterns of culture, for conscience "has taught a few of us to stand up for human dignity and rights in the face of the heaviest odds."[15] Similarly, Martin Luther King, Jr., in his "Letter from a Birmingham Jail," appealed to conscience as a challenge to positive law— but only because he could appeal to a more universal law that transcended individual societies: "How does one determine whether a law is just or unjust? A just law is a man-made code that squares with the moral law or the law of God. An unjust law is a code that is out of harmony with the moral law. To put it in the terms of St. Thomas Aquinas: 'An unjust law is a human law that is not rooted in eternal law and natural law.'"[16] Finally, consider Franz Jagerstatter, an Austrian villager who refused to fight for Hitler, insisting that his church and national leaders were repressing the very data that months before they acknowledged. All three of these people of conscience were the opposite of relativists or subjectivists, although they were preeminently personalists. Their challenges were made in the name of a value that transcended culture.[17]

This dimension of "objectivity" in moral judgments sustains and supports the human capacity to resist any customary morality that has enthroned the values of a select group as absolute. Customary morality, whether blindly accepted or highly rationalized, grounds itself in the mores of the group: one's family, one's nation, one's tribe. Thus, some people will propose "my country right or wrong" as their basic ethical standard. Others will fall back on the positive law of the state, or "whatever the party dictates," or whatever the majority thinks. These forms of cultural relativism can be challenged, however, only if there is a foundation for ethics other than the heritage one finds oneself lodged in.

When I was teaching for a year in Zimbabwe, many of the young men were being brought up with the cultural practice of *lobola* found in some of their ethnic communities. In this tradition, would-be grooms pay the family of the future bride for the privilege of marriage. One can assume that it had some economic, social, and political value for the community (quite possibly, one might suspect, especially for the males).

Some marriage processions would be halted right in the middle of the road with the bride being forced by parents or brothers to sit until the groom would promise more money.

The effects of this practice on families, children, and especially women were appalling. One student recalled his mother being beaten continually by her husband; his justification was, "I paid for you." Another student reported that infertile men could blame their wives for barrenness and send them back to their families in shame.

The quandary was this: It was always done. It was defended as socially necessary. It was accepted. "It is our way, and outsiders do not have a right to propose otherwise."[18]

The students, however, needed no outsider to prime their moral judgment. They had always judged it to be wrong. Their problem was in executing their moral judgment, their conscience. In our discussions concerning human dignity and human rights, it was evident to them that women, in every way, qualify as human persons. In the *lobola*, however, women were not treated as such. They were treated as property. The more morally sound of these young men decided to resist the practice.

NEGATION OF TRUTH AND THE BEGINNING OF EVIL

Underneath systems of racism, oppression, and sexual exploitation lie the fundamental dynamics of moral evil. Evil is a rejection of the truth of who and what we are as persons. It is a repression of evidence that points to our truth. It is a denial of ethics itself, grounded in the reality of personhood. Evil is a repudiation of conscience.

The very exercise of my self-defining activities and choices is not only the unique revelation of my personal existence. It is an implicit but necessary affirmation of the reality of personhood. Any moment of ethical decision requires the affirmation of personal reality as ethical reality.

To do ethics, to place an ethical act, is to tacitly affirm personal existence. It is to say "yes" to the human event of rationality and freedom in time. It is to confirm the truth of our embodied self-consciousness as persons. We cannot "do" ethics or "be" ethical if at the same time we negate personal existence. Our very impulse to be ethical, to be morally outraged, to be free, is an implicit demand for the affirmation of personal reality.

To some extent, this position is similar to Kant's second formulation of his categorical imperative: never to reduce a moral agent or person to the condition of being a mere thing. My argument here, however, is not based on the logic of moral consciousness alone (if one construes Kant in this standard—perhaps too narrow—fashion). It is based on the historically concrete men and women who bring ethics into the world. It is not based on a theoretical system. It is based on personhood. The voiding of persons is not merely a violation of moral logic. It is a rejection of the existential order—and of ethics itself.

To negate personhood, to deny its reality, to repress its moral truth, is the foundational negation of all ethics. To reduce men and women to the condition of replaceable and expendable objects is to deny their reality and to deny the foundation of the ethical impulse. It is the primary ethical negation. It is the primordial ethical rejection.

Thus, the positive formulation of the primary law of all ethical behavior is this: Affirm the reality of personal existence. Less abstractly, it requires the love of persons and the love of personal existence, for all love is the affirmation of the truth of the beloved as being good.

The negative formulation is this: Do not treat persons as nonpersons. Do not reduce persons to the status of an object.

The very intelligibility of ethics and ethical action rests on the confirmation of the fact that the human person is irreplaceable as a moral event, as a unique freedom capacitated for self-ownership in moral action. Ethics requires a recognition of the inherent moral value of persons and the intrinsic dignity of persons.

There is ethics, there is freedom, there is love, only because there are men and women in the world. One cannot affirm this truth, one cannot affirm ethics, in any act that negates or represses the person.

This view of human personhood is profoundly exalted. It carries with it, however, a crucial moral constraint on my behavior in the world. If I am to be ethically good and right, I am radically obliged to perform activities that do not negate or repress the intrinsic value of any human person.

Resistance to this limit and repression of the fundamental moral truth of our existence as persons is carried out in the name of countless secondary truths and values. Some of us will do it for nation, some for privilege. Some of us will do it for power, others for fame or pleasure. In all cases, however, we will find an absolute refusal to submit to the intrinsic value of persons.

FALLS AND CRIMES

One of the most harrowing portrayals of this moral refusal appears in Albert Camus' *The Fall.*[19] Jean-Baptiste Clamence, the inverted John the Baptist, announces not redemption but the second "fall" of humanity. He is a voice crying in the wilderness of a rotting Europe where men and women are mere silhouettes interested only in ideas, fornication, and newspapers. His endless monologue—an appropriate novel form for the underlying message—reveals that he is a human of complete deception and denial. Although this monologue seemingly is triggered by a failure to respond to a drowning voice calling for help in the night, his repression of truth penetrates his being. Not only must he deny his moral failure; he must deny that it made any difference. He is, admittedly, "two-faced," "a play-actor," a "liar." Utterly devoted to the fundamental fraudulence of the human being, he mutters that "truth is a colossal bore."[20]

> I have accepted duplicity instead of being upset about it. On the contrary, I have settled into it and found there the comfort I was looking for throughout life. I was wrong after all, to tell you that the essential was to avoid judgment. The essential is being able to permit oneself everything.[21]

In Clamence's case, his radical deception is not in the name of nation or money but his own ego—a value he holds so absolutely that he must repress the value of anything else, especially other egos. Camus portrays the "fall" of a man who permits and pardons himself to deny the intrinsic value of any person who might call him to judgment or make a claim on his life. Thus, he lies. He betrays friends. He uses and abuses women. He is racist. Especially, he is violent. He realizes that the nature of all violence is its intent to reduce the other person to the condition of a mere object or at least a slave. "Everyman needs slaves as he needs fresh air. Commanding is breathing—you agree with me?"[22]

Clamence's goal, in effect, is to have no moral limits on his ego and his desire for self-satisfaction. Therefore he must not only deny the intrinsic value of persons: He must eliminate their personal reality as a threat to his imperial self.

> I could live happily only on the condition that all the individuals on earth, or the greatest possible number, were turned toward me, eternally

in suspense, devoid of independent life and ready to answer my call at any moment, doomed in short to sterility until the day I should deign to favor them. In short, for me to live happily it was essential for the creatures I chose not to live at all. They must receive their life, sporadically, only at my bidding.[23]

Clamence's absolutized ego demands a negation of the value of others. The only people he can really love, he says, are dead ones. For if they are alive, the truth of their existence and value would be a rebuke to his dominion. "I pity without absolving, I understand without forgiving, and above all, I feel at last that I am being adored."[24]

Clamence, we might think, surely is a bizarre and extreme case of human malice. Camus invites us into his character with subtlety, however, so that we can see ourselves, sometimes even in our most ordinary pretenses and infidelities. Denial and deception are Clamence's very being. They also may be our commonplace tactics. Clamence's ego is so massive, it dwarfs all other realities. Every time we use a person, that person becomes a mere satellite of our desires. In the end, Camus requires us to ask of ourselves: Is all of our moral failure related to the covert wish to be adored?

Far less grand in scope but more recent and, perhaps, more telling is Woody Allen's film *Crimes and Misdemeanors*. It is peopled by a cast of liars: a self-infatuated TV producer (played by Alan Alda) who wants a fabricated film biography of himself; the Woody Allen character, Clifford, who deludes himself about his relationships and his integrity; a "life-affirming" philosophy professor who mouths words of love and then shoots himself; Mia Farrow's Holly, who protests that the producer is an obnoxious creep and then marries him; Jack Rosenthal, a professional thief and killer who has made deception his life.[25]

The central character is Doctor Judah Rosenthal—husband, father, modest golfer, respected civic leader, and ophthalmologist—who is also Jack's brother. Judah happens to be at the end of a tiring relationship with his mistress, an airline hostess named Dolores (played by Angelica Houston). The long-suffering Dolores, however, "going through hell," is not willing to give up the affair. In her brokenness, she is somewhat honest, and she threatens to bring the affair to the attention of Judah's wife.

Terrified by the possibility of disclosure and the danger to his profession and marriage ("I will not be destroyed by this woman"), Judah turns to two people for advice. The first is a rabbi, seemingly the only truthful person in the film, now going blind and a patient of Judah. He recommends honesty and openness and the possibility of forgiveness. The second is Jack, Judah's brother.

When Jack recommends "getting rid" of the problem by getting rid of Dolores, Judah is at first revulsed. "I can't believe we're talking like this about a human being. She's not an insect. You just can't stomp on her." Jack, however, reminds Judah that Dolores is the kind of person who will not be missed, a person whose death will bring about the best results for everyone. Jack chides his brother for his inability to face the "real world." As Jack says later, "Morality is a luxury I can't afford."

In a series of flashbacks to Judah's childhood, his father is the pre-vision of the blind rabbi, articulating a vision of the world as created with a moral structure and seen by a transcendent God. Judah's aunt, rendered cynical by the abominations of the Holocaust, maintains that there is no right or wrong other than the exercise of power; she is a pre-figuring of Jack's "realism": "If he can do it and chooses not to worry about the ethics, he can get away with it."

When the pressure from his mistress becomes unbearable, Judah finally calls Jack to have the killing done. Dolores is easily disposed of by an out-of-town hit man. She will not be missed. Judah will not be accused.

When Judah hears by telephone that the deed has been done, however, he is overcome by a sense of guilt and grief. He leaves his own celebration party to inspect the apartment of his mistress and is horrified by her empty eyes, the "eyes of the soul," as she once said—human but dead eyes that remind him of the "eyes of God seeing all" and the eyes of the rabbi, now empty in blindness.

Judah's guilt eventually wanes. He is fully convinced of the evil of his murder, but he learns to go on living. His crime is never discovered. It is never seen. He has "accepted the duplicity." At the end of the film, Judah finally has become comfortable with his enormous deception. The suicide-philosopher is quoted to the effect that we are defined by the choices we make.

Judah's choice was consciously in violation of his most fundamental convictions and moral judgments. Like any of us who might choose to extinguish a human life on behalf of quite laudable goals, he refused to accept the demands of a moral universe. The truth of one human being's value and existence was successfully repressed. The truth of her murder was as well.

And—he got away with it. It's the real world.

Like Judah, we might be appalled at first by the thought of killing an innocent person. Also like him, however, we may have our reasons. He murdered to save his career, his marriage, his property, his future.

Might we have our reasons? My home? My family? My livelihood? My land? My religion? A desperate desire? Fame? Love? Crack? Respect? Righteousness?

Are there no limits to what we might do, provided the cause is compelling enough?

7

Killing Persons and Ethics

A moral for doctors. The sick man is a parasite of society. In certain cases, it is indecent to go on living. To continue to vegetate in a state of cowardly dependence upon doctors and special treatments, once the meaning of life, the right to live has been lost, ought to be regarded with the greatest contempt by society. The doctors, for their part, should be agents for imparting this contempt—they should no longer prepare prescription, but should every day administer a fresh dose of *disgust* to their patients. A new responsibility should be created, that of the doctor—the responsibility of ruthlessly suppressing and eliminating *degenerate* life, in all cases in which the highest interests of life itself, of ascending life, demand such a course.

Friedrich Nietzsche[1]

We were told that my older brother, Theoneste Rukwirwa . . . had to be killed in order to prove that the whole family were not agents. . . . He himself brought the hoe and handed it to me. I hit him on the head. I kept hitting him on the head but he would not die. It was agonizing. Finally, I took the machete he dreaded in order to finish him off quickly. The [enemy] were there during the whole time, supervising what they called "work." They said that Theoneste had to die so the rest of us could live.

African Rights[2]

In regarding a newborn infant as not having the same right to life as a person, the cultures that practised infanticide were on solid ground.

Peter Singer[3]

Inevitably, part of good "orchestration" of a patient's last days may require euthanasia or assisted suicide.

Erich H. Loewy[4]

113

The history of the 20th century can be read as a catalogue of expendable people. Armenians, Hindus, Muslims, Christians, Aboriginal peoples, Africans, Afrikaaners, Jews, Lebanese, Palestinians, American Blacks, White Russians, Serbians, Vietnamese, Cambodians, Tibetans, Nicaraguans, Argentines, Mestizos, East Timorese, Algerians, Cubans, Bosnians, Rwandans, and Chinese have all seen themselves placed upon the victim's altar: a slaughtering-block of history.

One might regard this litany as evidence for the undeniable insignificance of human life, the hatefulness of human nature, and the incorrigible tendency of humans to turn on each other for the sake of advantage, power, and comfort. Nietzsche, who has become a favorite of some contemporary academics, also was the philosophical harbinger of attitudes found in arrogant nations and euthanizing doctors. The "cold-bloodedness of murder with a good conscience," which he recommended for the battlefield in *Human, All Too Human,* has been extended, as he hoped, to the field of medicine in its treatment of "degenerate life," whether newly born or nearly dead.[5]

On the other hand, one also might regard the history of ruthless violence as evidence for the undeniable fact of moral evil in the world—the cost of human freedom—wherein men and women choose to negate the fundamental moral limit of our lives by willing the extermination of the "other."

Perhaps most telling would be to interpret the violence of humanity upon itself as a spectrum of *justifications* for killing, as a litany of *exceptions* for choosing to extinguish human life. Every perpetrator of every outrage has had good reasons and important causes for every death: to defend my life, my name, my property, my family, my heritage, my race, my nation, my religion. In each case, some moral "absolute" often is invoked—but never the absolute value of a human life. Instead (as I show shortly), the absolute claim of some *other* interest that allows the killer an *exceptionalism* unites the logic of the terrorist with the logic of the respectable nation.

In this chapter, I reflect on the phenomenon of intentional killing of human beings. Because I propose a principle of total prohibition as the foundational moral command, I first review a range of reasons for killing persons, with the underlying strategies of justification and dehumanization. Then I suggest how the same strategies are used in two major medical controversies: abortion and physician-assisted suicide. As responses to the questions "Who count as persons and may we kill them?" I offer the following: Human persons are embodied careers, endowed with reflexive consciousness, and they may never be killed intentionally.

THE LOGIC OF TERROR

As 1998 began, a New York courtroom was the scene of a rare but harrowing moment of truth. Ramzi Ahmed Yousef, the Iraqi mastermind of the 1997 World Trade Center bombing, just sentenced to 240 years in prison, admitted he was a terrorist, "and I am proud of it." The judge called Yousef an "apostle of evil" who killed for the thrill of killing (a sentiment shared by most Americans). The terrorist, however, had a different perspective:

> You keep talking about collective punishment and killing innocent people to force governments to change their policies. . . . You call this terrorism. . . . Well, you were the first ones who invented this terrorism . . . when you dropped an atomic bomb which killed tens of thousands of women and children in Japan. . . . You killed them by burning them to death. You killed civilians in Vietnam with chemicals. . . . You went to wars more than any other country in this century, and then you have the nerve to talk about killing innocent people.
>
> And now you have new ways to kill the innocent. You have so-called economic embargo which kills nobody other than children and elderly people. . . . Yes, I am a terrorist, and I am proud of it. And I support terrorism so long as it is against the United States and Israel because you are more than terrorists. You are the ones who invented it . . . butchers, liars, and hypocrites.[6]

Did Yousef have a point? The United States' official position had been that the terror of bombs was the one language that Saddam understood. Innocents might suffer, but only as impersonal "collateral damage." Such is the very argument Yousef used against us, however: "This is what it takes to make you feel the pain which you are causing to other people."

The foregoing comparison is not intended to make a case for Yousef. The United States was not the first nation to use the logic of terror. Furthermore, Yousef seems utterly incapable of acknowledging the malice of his own leader. Yet he understands well our justifications for the terror we work on others. He reveals the deadly rationale we employ not only for sanctions against his people but for our claim to have the "right to unilaterally bomb Iraq." Moreover, he is living proof that any humiliation and destruction we may rain on Saddam Hussein and his people will only confirm his hatred for us and our moral posturing.

News magazines reported after Operation Desert Storm that the few Iraqis willing to speak to Americans had only anxious questions: Will we be bombed again? Why us? Haven't we suffered enough? These people have lived with a history of colonialism and Western interference. Their city was sprayed with 88,000 tons of bombs in 100,000 raids by the United States during the Gulf War. Since then, civilians— mostly infants—have suffered from the destruction of Baghdad's capacity to deliver clean water, good food, and effective medical care.[7]

When children were killed as the result of American bombing, our leaders claimed that such casualties were Saddam's fault because he held them hostage near strategic targets. Suppose, however, that all our presumptions are true—that his people are not with him, that they want liberation, that they are unwilling pawns; we still must ask ourselves a question: If a mad killer surrounds himself with children, do we shoot through their bodies to stop his terror? If we do so, we embrace his own ruthless logic. We will understand more intimately why Hutus could kill innocent Tutsis, why the roads of Bosnia run with blood, why Cambodia still reels from the whirl of deadly force.

I am not speaking of the moral equivalence of persons here. No doubt, many Iraqis would resent such comparisons—as most Americans, for different reasons, would. I am speaking of the equivalence of moral reasoning, or the lack of it. To bomb Iraq is to perpetuate the logic of the terrorist Yousef and the moral chaos he represents. It is to succumb to the fatal rationalizing that makes persons expendable for the sake of a supposedly higher goal.

A refusal to bomb persons does not leave a nation helpless. There are economic and political strategies available for those who challenge unjust power. There also are strategic *admissions* that the United States, like any nation, might make. After all, we produce weapons—more than any people in history; many of them are designed to kill populations, by chemical or explosive means. We also sell weapons that are used by both sides of every war. Likewise, we threaten people. In fact, in Yousef's eyes, that is what we were doing to Iraq. U.S. policy also helped make Saddam Hussein what he became. He was "our boy" when he fought Iran in the 1980s. We ignored his murder of the Kurds. We regarded his oil, and the oil of other OPEC countries, as our strategic resource, the loss of which would endanger "our way of life." Any examination of conscience over matters of the Middle East, of Lebanon, of cheap petroleum, of proxy governments, of orchestrated coups, might lead us to see why some people think we are part of the problem.

That would be a start. Then we must let go of our nonnegotiable and one-sided demands. After all, would we allow an Iraqi-controlled United Nations to inspect our munitions and bases? Would we be inclined to forgive the aerial bombing of New York's infrastructure? Unlikely, judging from our outrage at the bombing of the World Trade Center. Judge Kevin Thomas Duffy, at the terrorist's trial, rightly turned his wrath on Yousef. "Your God is death. Your God is not Allah. . . . You worship death and destruction. What you do, you do only to satisfy your own twisted sense of ego." The question to be raised for us all, however, is whether we, too—when we are as "justified" in our killing as Yousef is—worship a god of death.

If we realized that the living God might not always be on our side, that all our wars might not be holy, we might be more fit to criticize Saddam Hussein and demand honest and honorable negotiations. Should that fail, economic pressure and political isolation can be applied not only to him but to those "most favored nations" for whose trade we compromise our principles. If he then attacks the innocent, those who believe in just wars might warrant invasion. Even then, I propose, we will be entertaining a most dangerous calculus of human expendability. If the United States once again decides to throw missiles at Iraq, then the terrorist Yousef will have won the debate. His logic of terror will have captured our hearts and minds once again.

The competing but complementary arguments of the United States versus Ramzi Yousef can be regarded as the upshot of all relativisms that install one's people, one's tribe, or one's nation as the basis of moral value. Ultimately, both arguments are grounded on the permissibility of killing for a good enough reason—usually *protecting* human lives, whether they are Yousef's people or our allies. The one principle we never appeal to, however, is the principle of the inviolability of personal existence. Because that would prohibit all intentional killing, it is the one principle we always negate.

The destruction we humans inflict on each other, especially in the extremes of individual or state terrorism, is a massive denial of the value of human existence in the name of more pressing desires. The tendency to absolutize any value *other* than the human person is so powerful, the resistance to any moral "limit" on the exercise of our imperial "choice" so strong, that even those who mouth the words of human dignity and human rights are driven to deny the humanity of other men and women so that killing them can be justified.

Non-Greeks were "barbarians"; non-Chinese were "foreign devils," Chinese were "gooks"; Germans were "huns," Jews were sub-human in the Nazi Primers given to Hitler Youth; criminals are vermin, fetuses are "blobs of protoplasm," terminally ill people are "vegetables"; Africans were "savages"; Communists were "monsters," capitalists were "pigs"; Margaret Thatcher was a "witch," the IRA were "immoral animals"; blacks and women were "property," Amerinds were "brutes." Dehumanization allows us to destroy any loathed object.

"One million Arabs are not worth a Jewish fingernail," proclaims a fanatical rabbi before a thousand sympathizers.[8] "Never will I say I am not an anti-Semite. I pray that God will kill my enemy and take him off the face of the planet earth," preaches an equally fanatical minister of the Nation of Islam.[9]

The terrible irony of these two quotations is that Yitzhak Rabin, who challenged the killing logic of Jews and Arabs, was assassinated by Yigal Amir, whose motive was to save Jews. The Amir Defense Line of Manhattan regards Amir as a hero: "We felt that this whole incident saved hundreds of thousands of Jewish lives. It was equivalent to somebody killing Adolf Hitler before the Holocaust."[10] The circle of killing continues, but only to "save" lives.

This is the ever-present strategy of rendering human beings expendable. In all the killings of history, the intrinsic value and moral dignity of the human person has always been repressed and denied. Instead, the secondary values or goods that *make* persons valuable have been affirmed. They were innocent, they were friendly, they were strategic, their lives were meaningful and productive, they were "wanted," they were fully functioning, they acted like a person, they were white and male, Christian, Jew, or Muslim, they were of the right caste or class. Thus, the guilty, the enemy, the alien, and the unwanted were candidates for elimination. In the mind of Yigal Amir, Yitzhak Rabin was expendable because he was "equivalent to . . . Adolf Hitler" and because killing Rabin would "save hundreds of thousands."

THE MORAL INVIOLABILITY OF PERSONS

There are entire libraries on the moral question of terminating human life.[11] Not many entries advocate the position I offer here: radical personalism. By "radical" I mean two things. This ethic is rooted in the very existence of personhood, which makes ethics possible and ultimately grounds any claims made for human rights or dignity. It also is radical in that it yields the root prohibition against the direct intentional killing of any human being.

As a treatment of foundations in ethics, this work concentrates on the founding principle that a personalist brings to any concrete issue of life and death. This moral principle is both direct and concise. It also is highly demanding as a moral standard. Most likely, that is why it has been rejected throughout history when men and women have found it more realistic to render others dispensable.

Because the very impulse to be ethical affirms the personal reality from which ethics springs—because the very placement of an ethical act is, of its essence, a "yes" to personal dignity—one cannot be faithful to the moral universe in doing any act that in itself negates personhood in oneself or another. Fidelity to human personhood, the affirmation of the intrinsic value of human persons and adherence to the truth of personal moral dignity, requires that we never reduce a human person to the condition of being a nonperson, that we not negate the personhood of our selves or others, that we not treat a person as a mere thing or object.

Because the most definitive and irreversible way to turn a person into a thing, to reduce a person to an object, to negate existing personal reality, is to kill a person, a personalist ethics requires an exceptionless prohibition against the intentional killing of a human being.

To be willing to kill a human person is to be willing to kill the foundation of ethics itself. It is to disengage oneself from the moral universe. There surely are greater and lesser evil acts of killing, but one quality that all such acts share is the willed extermination of personal life. A deliberate killing is the consciously known and willed negation of human personhood. It literally turns a person into a thing. It is an ultimate renunciation of personal existence, an irrevocable repression of the truth of what we are.

The intent to kill is crucial here. Killing can be nonintentional and thereby premoral. Killing also may have purportedly further evil motives and purposes, which would likely qualify it as murder in some legal context. The intent to kill persons, however, is itself a radical compromise of moral life. So deep is this consciousness in us that we must inevitably rationalize the killing of persons, repress their personhood, or deaden our own primal ethical sensibilities. As David Grossman has recounted in *On Killing: The Psychological Cost of Learning to Kill in War and Society*, if efforts to construe the enemy as "less than an animal" or "an inferior form of life" do not work, the psychological toll is horrific:

> Killing is the worst thing that one man can do to another man. . . . It's the last thing that should happen anywhere. (Israeli lieutenant)

> I reproached myself as a destroyer. An incredible uneasiness came over me. I felt almost like a criminal. (Napoleonic-era British soldier)

> This was the first time I had killed anybody and when things quieted down I went and looked at a German I knew I had shot. I remember thinking that he looked old enough to have a family and I felt very sorry. (British World War I veteran, after his first kill)

> It didn't hit me all that much then, but when I think of it now—I slaughtered those people. I murdered them. (German World War II veteran)

> I just opened up, fired the whole 20 rounds right at the kid, and he just laid there. I dropped my weapon and cried. (U.S. Special Forces officer in Vietnam)[12]

The prohibition against killing persons is the limit situation in ethics. It is the ultimate constraint on all exercise of autonomy because the very appeal to autonomy is an appeal to the dignity of personhood. If we violate this principle, we violate the moral order and the claims that personal reality make on us. This is not to say that torture, brainwashing, and slavery are less evil. It is to say that such cruelty partakes in the fundamental depersonalization of which intentional killing is the prime, irreversible example. An ethics of radical personalism yields to the exceptionless moral principle that personal life must not be negated—because in doing so, the foundation of moral experience itself is rejected.

Radical personalism makes the following contentions:

- Human dignity is objective—undiminished by special situations, extrinsic relativities or interior dispositions.

- The demand to defend ourselves, our family, or our nation is rooted *not* in the narcissist particularity of *our* nation, family, desires, or goals but in the universal experience of personal dignity.
- Every issue of "beneficence" or "care" or "informed consent" or "autonomy" in medical ethics has its meaning *only if there are beings in the world called human*, endowed with intrinsic capacities and invested with intrinsic moral value.[13]
- Every legal or international issue of rights or equality, of fairness or injustice, of property or retribution, is founded on the reality of human personhood.
- Every discussion of "happiness" for the greatest number or "obligation" for the individual is rooted in the phenomenon of humanity.

On this account, the value of a human being is intrinsic. It is not a function of being American or Iraqi, Israeli or Palestinian. Your intrinsic value does not cease if you feel meaningless or suffer pain. It does not end if you are no longer young or attractive. It does not cease when you are comatose or drunk or imprisoned. It is not based on your actions, your functioning, your achievement, or your failure, even if you are a murderer yourself. Your intrinsic value does not begin when you are wanted or approved. It does not start when you are recognized by the state. It is not "bestowed" on you when you start breathing or talking or acting responsibly.

Intrinsic personal value—the foundation of ethical value—starts when our individual life journeys begin. It ends only with the cessation of our existence.

Therefore the investigation concerning what *makes* us human and who *counts* as human is crucial. The human person is an embodied, reflexively conscious career. As bodies, we are developing, unfolding realities, with physical endowments that are actualized at various stages in the drama of our lives. Because we are endowed with reflexive consciousness, the range of our human career provides the opportunity to exercise this capacity in freedom, intelligent creativity, loving action, and moral choice.

Personal endowments are "gifts" by reason of our humanity, not gifts of the state or society or others or even time itself—although these conditions surely are required for the actualization and fulfillment of these gifts. Without the cultivation of family, culture, and other relations, we would never be realized as persons and selves. We couldn't do that without air or food as well.

These preeminently personal endowments are the basis of our radical equality: The gift of our humanness is the same in every human. Our *inequalities* are not a function of our common humanity and its endowments; they are a function of the differences wherein our endowments are actualized and nurtured within our various organic conditions and the influences of diverse environments. How, where, and why we develop these endowments is also why we are each personally unique. Each human history and context, providing the stage for our personal life-narrative, is the occasion for a person's original and irreplaceable "yes."

Moreover, these endowments are real, even though they may not be actualized. We were human persons long before we started to act like mature persons. From the moment we began, each of us started as a certain "kind" of being, launched on a career of self-development and self-expression. Damage, deprivation, or lack of development may shorten or debilitate our careers, but they are careers of human persons and not something else. The existential reality of a person is not the same as the activities of a person or the varying fulfillments that person experiences.

These observations are worth further formulation because the foundational ethical principle of a radical personalism is directly related to criteria we have for acknowledging a human person and determining when a human's life begins and ends. The founding law of a personalist ethics legislates that we be faithful to human personhood, faithful to its constitution in us and in others, faithful to its value as it is embodied in existing persons.

DEFENDING LIFE BY INTENDING DEATH

The main objection to a nonkilling principle has involved the threat of an unjust aggressor. May I, my family, or my nation do nothing if our own lives are at stake? Does this principle not degrade our own value as persons?

A radical personalist can respond that defending ourselves is a positive moral good. Even more, we may do everything in our power to defend ourselves—*short* of violating the foundational principle itself by intending to kill personal life. Aggression does not make the aggressor a nonperson. In fact, most of the atrocities committed against the groups mentioned at the beginning of this chapter were "justified" as a defense against real or imagined aggressors.

The deliberate will to kill a human is crucial here. The intent is one with the choice. A peace officer might shoot to stop or wound a criminal and accidentally kill the offender. That is undeniably different than someone following out or privately assuming a "shoot-to-kill" policy. The consequential results are not the sole determinant of the quality of the moral act; the intent is equally significant as descriptive of the moral act itself. Thus, an assassin who intends to kill violates the moral order, even if the plans for murder fail in the execution. Police officers routinely intend to stop an aggressor. Sometimes they accidentally kill the aggressor. This distinction is as crucial as it is a test of one's honesty. It is crucial because we constantly choose courses of action that have unintended results. It is a test of one's honesty because no one but ourselves can examine our intent.

The principle of nonkilling is not a recommendation of passivity. To the contrary: A primary commitment to the inherent dignity of personal life *requires* us to intervene on behalf of the defenseless or the victim. Our only moral limit is the direct intended killing of the aggressor.

A *lack* of commitment to intrinsic personal dignity allowed people to stand by passively not only when Hitler came to power but also while he destroyed millions. Hitler exploited the rationale of self-defense to justify his own outrages. Most of his followers swallowed his rationalization. There were no editorialists and few ethicists in Frankfurt, Berlin, or Munich who proposed that Germany was mounting an unjust war. We readily imagine what we might have done to resist Hitler. The tougher question, however, involves what we would have done if he were on *our* side. The thousands of conscientious objectors during the Vietnam War who were taunted with the question: "Would you have fought against Hitler?" should have responded, "Would you have fought *for* him?"

Has there ever been a war that was not justified by both sides? Has there ever been an assassination or act of terrorism that has not been rationalized by some logic of self-defense? Even the horrors of Rwanda used such perverse justification.

> "When you are killing the wives, don't spare those who are pregnant. The mistake we made in 1959 was not to kill the children. Now they have come back to fight us. . . ."

"They said my godmother was a Tutsi and therefore I was also a Tutsi. They said I must kill my godmother. They began to insist and started beating me up. When I felt that the beating was too much, I gave in and hit my godmother with the machete. . . ."

"Either you kill them, or you will be killed. . . ."

"A Hutu man who had four children with a Tutsi wife was forced to kill two of the children who were considered to have the mother's Tutsi looks. . . ."

"Everybody [including children] was killed, because if one escaped, he could come back to attack us. . . ."

"I regret what I did. . . . I am ashamed, but what would you have done if you had been in my place? Either you took part in the massacre or else you were massacred yourself."[14]

We should note that many Hutus and Tutsis heroically resisted the maelstrom of rationalized evil. Some paid the ultimate price—their lives and the lives of their families—for their solidarity with the demonized "other." The reason the killing reached such massive proportions, however, was the deadly logic—albeit illusory—of self-defense and survival. Neighbors killed neighbors and their children because, if they did not, everything they held dear, including their lives, would be lost. In survival, conscience and ethics itself were lost.

The Rwandan tragedy pushes the argument of self-defense to the limit. It also suggests the awesome threshold one crosses when one rationally justifies intentional killing for the sake of life. There are indeed significant moral differences between noble warriors and ignoble ones. There also is one crucially significant principle they share: Given the right conditions, the appropriate act is extinction of a human being. Perhaps, as Thomas Nagel has written, "The world can present us with situations in which there is no honorable or moral course for a man to take, no course free of guilt and responsibility for evil."[15] If the killing of persons is one of those situations, Nagel's expression is apt. It is a suspension of the moral universe. Once one has left that universe, one is easily led to consider the terror bombings of Dresden and London, the burned children of Nagasaki and Shanghai, the mass graves of Leningrad and Auschwitz, and the ashes of Lebanon—the unfortunately required costs of defending ourselves and our innocents.[16]

This moral logic has justified the violence of the late 20th century: in the rape and pillage of Yugoslavia and Kosovo, in the splinters of the Soviet Union, in the forced starvations of Somalia and Sudan, in the bombings of Iraq and Tripoli, in the U.S. support of contras to overthrow Nicaragua's government and the U.S. support of El Salvador's military to prop up a tyranny, in the "necklacing" by the Inkatha and the hymns to AK-47s by the African National Congress and the invocation of holy scriptures by Afrikaaners. It is the excuse of fundamentalists in Texas and Teheran, the explanation of liberals in New York and conservatives in London, the justification of those who kill abortion doctors, the apologia of Parisian leftists pardoning the atrocities of Mao and Stalin.

Such logic also is a justification for capital punishment, the most deliberate and ornate termination of human existence—especially in a land where secure pundits and scared politicians explain the act as "respect for human life."[17]

The destruction of personal existence is closest to each of us in advanced industrial technologies in the area of medical ethics, however. The killing of marginal, damaged, or unfinished human beings has been offered to us as the most highly rationalized, socially acceptable, and culturally strategic form of extinguishing personhood. In controversies concerning the beginning and the ending of a human's life, the phenomena of depersonalization and human devaluation mark public discourse and national policy.

KILLING INCOMPLETE PERSONS

In ethical issues that involve the earliest and the last stages of life, the central question for the personalist is *whether* a human person is involved. Yet people often avoid this very question when they choose to terminate humans they consider unfinished, unwanted, or damaged. Either the candidate for killing is considered less than human, or the data that refute such a claim is ignored.

With regard to termination of pregnancies, the endowment theory of personalism holds that whenever a human life begins, an individual person has started on a human career. This issue—whether we are dealing with a human person or not—is different from the issue of whether one may kill humans. Even if we are dealing with a human being, some people hold that, under certain conditions, the termination of a human life is ethically permissible. These conditions might include guilt as opposed to innocence, foe as opposed to friend, or—in the case of many medical issues—severe pain, meaninglessness, lack of development, profound disability, social threat, and so forth. None of these exceptions would be allowed by the principle of the exceptionless inviolability of persons.

Be that as it may, one must be aware of the evidence to which people might point in indicating the moment at which a human person is present. Several possibilities have been propounded.

Fertilization or conception is the first stage at which a human person might be present. The evidence for this claim is the fact that at that moment, a unique, genetically endowed life is launched. The embodied individual now known as you or me began with endowments, physical and otherwise. Although these endowments require time to be actualized, they are nonetheless present and real—as real as the fact that I am male rather than female. My maleness or femaleness began, long before the formation of my brain or any primary and secondary sexual characteristics. The zygote is a radically different kind of being than a sperm or ovum—neither of which has any internal principle of self-development or elaboration. A sperm may have the endowments to enter into a new unique union with an ovum, but it is not a humanly endowed career. Once conception has taken place, however, the career of this human person can be profoundly changed by genetic intervention. In such a case, the person's life and being is changed. This account of human personhood, consequently, gives full weight to the fact that we are biological beings, ontologically individual, naturally endowed. Personhood is not a function of performance or actualized capacities; it is a function of the kind of being we are.[18]

A second stage that might suggest the beginning of a single unique human career occurs once twinning or recombination is no longer possible. Up to the 13th day, the conceived being may appear to be operating as a number of related processes, but not one individual. The cells are "totipotential," rather than differentiated as parts of one integrated organism. Thus, they are capable of division into separate units. Sometime between the 13th and 20th days, twinning can still take place. Although such twinning likely is programmed from conception by the RNA of the mother, many people suggest that a unique individual has not irreversibly started until after this time. If a person must be onto-logically an individual being with one life, the embryonic stage called the "primitive streak" seems most appropriate as the moment of a new integration and organic unity called a human career.[19] Data concerning this stage are important in controversies concerning "morning-after" pills, preimplantation diagnosis, and "stem-cell" research.

The late astrophysicist Carl Sagan agreed with the theory of bioethicist Baruch Brody that a human person does not exist until there is a brain. On approximately the 20th day after conception, the gradual formation of a precortex gets underway. By the 40th to 43rd day, there is identifiable brain activity, detectable by an EEG. Sagan wrote in pop-ular publications that by 6–8 weeks we should somehow protect the un-born as a human person. The endowment theory, on the other hand, holds that the human person is capacitated to *develop* a brain but is not *re-ducible* to the brain, its development, or its damage. As Eric Olson has pointed out in *The Human Animal: Personal Identity Without Psychology*, mak-ing a functioning brain the crucial requirement for personhood is a con-temporary rendition of "brain-state" Cartesianism that does not take our organic life seriously. (Oddly enough, it also would preempt the possi-bility that there could be other kinds of persons besides humans with brains.) Other emphases on actualized capacities—for example, heart-beat, sonogram representations, the experience of "quickening," or fetal movement—also have been proposed as functional or performance cri-teria, rather than intrinsic endowments.[20]

The Supreme Court decision in *Roe v. Wade* suggested that some-thing significant happens at the third trimester, meriting a different set of legal constraints that the various states might impose upon abortion procedures. This approach seems to be related to a "viability" criterion—which itself has significantly shifted over the past 30 years with new developments in neonatal technology. It suffers from the fact that, in principle, with the possibility of artificial wombs, a conceptus might be "viable" from the start.

Finally, some people seem to think that a human person doesn't ac-tually begin until birth—or even some time after. Certain criteria—such as bonding, wantedness, conscious desires, or good brain functioning—determine personhood "status." Although the newborn child of a man and woman, on this account, is surely an "animal" and a human, it is not a person. This approach seems to require that personhood has neither ontological status nor biological grounding; instead, it is something bestowed on us by others or suddenly emergent when certain actions are performed.[21]

Among the crucial issues that surface in the abortion debate, a woman's autonomy and control over her reproductive life must be given a prominent place. Undeniably, there is weighty historical evidence that women have been unjustly deprived of personal liberty, especially in their sexual lives. The preeminent issue here, however, is that if abortion involves two human persons (albeit at different stages of a personal career) rather than one, autonomy does not override and cannot negate the intrinsic value of a person. Such is the personalist position in any issue relating to termination of human existence.

Even if there were consensus, based on genetic and embryological evidence, that the career of an individual human person starts at the earliest stages of pregnancy, the personalist must confront a plurality of positions on the moral acceptability of intentional killing. Whether we are dealing with human persons in the womb or at infancy, maturity, or diminishment, is the intentional killing of them ethically permissible?

The possibilities are as follows:

- Yes, sometimes, *for a good reason* (rape, health, danger, self-defense)—just as there are reasons for killing persons in other situations: in war, as capital punishment, by physician-assisted suicide. In more extreme cases, some people might think killing anyone, guilty or innocent, is permissible for the sake of a desirable end (e.g., nation, family, property, one's well-being).
- Never an *innocent* life: Killing unjust aggressors is legitimate, as in war or capital punishment, but not abortion (unless, as some people hold, the human fetus can be seen as a threat or a danger to life, livelihood, well-being, etc.).
- *Never*: The position that allows no exception to the inviolability principle. This position prohibits all intentional killing of human persons, whether in capital punishment, just war, self-defense, euthanasia, or the abortion of a human.

The personalist position, in conjunction with the human endowment theory, maintains that intentionally killing another person is never permissible. This position, to be sure, is a minority position in contemporary life. Most troubling for the personalist, however, is the suggestion that the intrinsic value of personal life, even at the *last stages* of fetal development, is not to be considered. The theoretical denial of personal status to third-trimester human fetuses, which has led thinkers such as Peter Singer and Mary Ann Warren to deny that status to newborns, is mirrored in the practical deliberations of a Congress that is incapable of offering any legal restraint on late-term abortions and in the increasingly common moral tragedies of our social world. Two concrete vignettes represent our contemporary moral contortions over early human life.

On the coldest night of 1993, a two-week-old baby was beaten and tossed into a Newark dumpster. The wind-chill factor—an apt metaphor for the coldness of a world that abuses its most defenseless—was 17 degrees below zero. The hypothermic baby was rescued by a parking lot attendant and turned over to authorities. The authorities were at a loss with regard to what the mother should be charged with. The next day, in New York City, a five-pound, hours-old baby was found in a gym bag. Some of the hospital people named him "Jim" after the bag that held his naked body.

Meanwhile, a dreadful Manhattan trial was going on. Rosa Rodriguez was telling the jury that her daughter was born with only one arm. The right arm had been cut off in a botched abortion attempt, the day before her daughter's birth. (Ms. Rodriguez had been eight months pregnant at the time.) Most telling, perhaps, is the mother's response when she was presented with the simple evidence of what kind of being had been aborted. "I saw that her right arm was missing. They asked me if I wanted to keep her, and I told them, 'Yes.'" Only the most systemic repression of evidence could, until that moment, repress her intuitive affirmation of the human person before her eyes. The "doctor," who had charged the woman $1,000 for the abortion, was tried for violating state law prohibiting abortions after the 24th week—not attempted homicide, not mayhem and amputation, but violating a state law.[22]

In this matter of early personal life, the question arises whether we have collaborated in blinding ourselves so much that we are unable to respond to the simplest, undeniable evidence of the senses. Our corporate sensibilities may well have become so deadened that even the most elementary feelings of compassion and protection we provide for force-fed calves, laboratory mice, or baby seals cannot be extended to unborn humans. If we announced that tomorrow a kitten would be treated the way some 20-week-old unborn humans are treated daily in clinics and hospitals, who could still the protests?

For a few "pro-choice" advocates, the value of the private choice is so absolutized that no restraint can be considered, not even in the name of values that they themselves supposedly champion. Not in the name of "informed consent." Not in the name of others' individual consciences. Not to insure the autonomy of health institutions that would betray their public trust and traditions. Not to have a waiting period so that a woman might make a more informed choice or investigate options that would enhance her freedom. Not to let a woman know clearly what is happening to her body. Not to let her family or partner enter her deliberation. Especially not to raise the question of whether we are terminating the life of a human being.

The question, "Are we eliminating persons with potentials, and not just potential persons?" is absent from most public discourse, other than to say that abortion is more a matter of feeling than evidence. The evidence that a fetus is at least a human being is for the most part suppressed or reduced to a "religious issue."

How, then, could Bernard Nathanson, who presided over 50,000 abortions, later change his moral judgment—not because of "religion" but because of the overwhelming clinical evidence he had been killing human beings? Carl Sagan—no formal believer—believed that brain development dictates the judgment that we have a human being at least at the eighth week of fetal development. Nat Hentoff, a nonreligious Jew, compares our treatment of the unborn with our treatment of all "marginal" humans, yet he is relegated to the status of a quaint exception.[23]

On the other hand, the repression of evidence is as prevalent for some "pro-lifers" as it is with "pro-choicers." For example, many people deplore second- and third-trimester abortions and yet cannot agree with the proposition that a one-week-old conceived human is fully a "human baby." Thus, they resent as dishonest much of the powerful pro-life argumentation—the pictures of aborted fetuses, the ultrasound films, the data about pain, the severed members of a body—that does not apply to the first trimester, much less the first two weeks of a pregnancy (when most pregnancies are terminated and most spontaneous abortions occur). They do not think yelling "you're killing your baby" is truthful. They also realize that when a woman is shown the actual evidence of a two-week pregnancy, she clearly sees no activities of a minute "baby." They also know that the tremendous number of spontaneous abortions during the first two weeks is dramatically different than the saline and D&C "procedures" of later trimesters.

Rhetoric has overridden the evidence. The hard work of evidence and education is neglected. Perhaps this neglect is because there is enough scientific evidence, with ethical implications, to suggest that there can be an honest and fair difference of opinion about the "humanity" of a human conceptus during the first two weeks of pregnancy.[24] "Pro-life" groups rarely allow such a possibility, however, even in discussions of efforts to protect unborn humans at *any* stage of development. If you propose that you might be able to get political consensus to protect the life of all second- and third-trimester unborn, some of them will call you a heartless killer.

My own position is this: Humans begin their lives when the process of conception is completed. That is when the "life" begins. That is when the personal existence of John Kavanaugh began. The strongest evidence for this position is genetic. Something radically new takes place when a human ovum is united with a human sperm. A complete and unique genotype with its own internal principle of self-development is created. It has its inherent system of information for the elaboration and development of its own capacities and endowments. The career of a human person is launched—a person with potentials, not a potential person.

Claiming that an isolated sperm or ovum has the same endowments is disingenuous, if not silly. Claiming that we do not know if a conceived human is a different "kind" of being than nonpersonal animals is even sillier.

The argument for conception also is supported by the common-sense insight that my voice, my maleness, my color blindness—all of which are of me—began at the moment my individual life began, with its own internal unifying and integrated dynamism for self-development, open to actualization and fulfillment only with the assistance and information of multiple environments.

The theory of personally endowed nature helps us see that a human being need not be activating his or her potentialities to be human. An unborn child, like a comatose grandmother, is not a "potential" human but a human with endowments—even though they may not be activated because of development or damage.[25]

You and I did not begin at quickening or birth or breath or sensing or speaking. We began when our entire life process was initiated and started developing as a dynamic unity.

Many people do not know this evidence or disagree with it in good faith. This disagreement usually relates to the very earliest stages of our development. The evidence after the first two weeks—and most assuredly after the first eight weeks—is compelling, however. Finding someone who is open to the data, yet denies that we are dealing with a human being (albeit not a baby or a grandfather) in the truest sense of the word, is difficult. What is morally bankrupt, however, in the social and political arena is if countless men and women, legitimized by law, are consciously terminating the life of a being they know is human. They may, in conscience, think it is ethically acceptable to do so; this belief only compounds the moral failure, however.

What is morally bankrupt as well is the unwillingness of many "pro-life" people to allow any room for disagreement in evaluating the evidence. Those who honestly disagree about the data concerning the first days after conception are ignored. Their offers to collaborate politically for the sake of the unborn *after* the first trimester—when consensus is clearly available—are rejected.

Those who hold that a human being is present at conception must realize that developing a compelling argument for the humanity status of the fertilized egg requires diligent effort. The argument is based not only on sophisticated medical and genetic data but also on philosophical arguments of Aristotle and Aquinas—both of whom are difficult to comprehend, and neither of whom came to conclusions that contemporary genetics supports.[26]

The position of a radical personalist demands that evidence be investigated to protect the inviolability of any human life, including a human life at the earliest moment of conception if the data warrant that conclusion. On the basis of this evidence, the moral judgment of men and women who are politically franchised or elected can change. If law and politics do not change, the same avenues of resistance that are open to those who oppose war or capital punishment are available.

KILLING DEFECTIVE OR DYING PERSONS

The repression of evidence in choices concerning the earliest stages of life shows up again in choices that deal with life's end. The question of whether someone "counts" as a person is strategic, to be sure. The process of dehumanizing the "enemy" is repeated in the process of dehumanizing the "degenerate," the "hopeless," the "vegetable."

The prevailing personal value for those who wish to terminate their own lives or the lives of others is, again, "choice"—or, as the courts frame it, "the liberty interest." There seems to be no moral limit on this value, other than Mill's proposal that personal sovereignty is restricted by the rights of others. With regard to our own bodies—even the killing of them—we must have unfettered freedom.

> A competent, terminally ill adult, having lived nearly the full measure of life, has a strong liberty interest in choosing a dignified and humane death, rather than being reduced at the end of his existence to a childlike state of helplessness, diapered, sedated, incontinent.[27]

These words of Judge Stephen Reinhardt of the U.S. Court of Appeals for the Ninth Circuit prodded me to try to recall just when my late uncle lost his "dignity." Although he was somewhat helpless, sedated, and slightly incontinent when he died, the moment of his indignity escapes me.

For the most part, contemporary use of the word "dignity," like that of related notions such as "value" and "worth," points either inward to certain subjective attitudes or outward to extrinsic standards of usefulness, productivity, or measurable achievement.

The *inward* focus emphasizes one's state of mind. What makes me feel that I have dignity? What values about myself do I hold? What do I consider worthwhile? In its extreme form, this subjective focus can lead me to the conclusion that if I *feel* worthless, I *am* worthless. Dignity, in this case, is a state of mind that can be achieved or lost, depending on how I feel about myself. This position is exemplified by the student who announced to a medical ethics class that he would rather have his life terminated than live "without dignity." When he was asked what condition might strip him of his dignity, he suggested that being incontinent and diapered would fill the bill. He agrees with the honorable Judge Reinhardt.

The *outward* focus evaluates a person or thing in terms of a relationship to someone or something else. Here I judge myself to have dignity or value if I possess something or if I am perceived as valuable by other persons, an institution, or a state. My dignity in this context is a function of my instrumentality. If I am useful, I am good. I am valuable. I have dignity. If I am wanted, I am worthwhile. If I am attractive or powerful, able to take care of myself, wealthy or clean, these extrinsic qualities guarantee my dignity.

When value or dignity are reduced to subjective attitudes or external qualities, a strange paradox may hit us: Nothing and no one is to be valued for its own sake. No one has dignity; we have only feelings or appearances of dignity. I am a hollow me. We are an empty us. Everything of value about us is either how useful we may be or how good we may feel about ourselves. Nothing is worthy of respect. Everything is to be used. We are faced with the painful recognition that there is no interior life, no intrinsic dignity in ourselves for which we might be grateful or that we might betray.

For the personalist, the value of human choice is ethically limited by the intrinsic and inviolable value of a human life. Thus, the extrinsic reasons one invokes when one chooses to terminate a person's life do not override the inherent value of personal existence. Usefulness, meaningfulness, even pain or suffering do not give us value. Our value is a function of our being.

That is why the judge's pronouncement on losing dignity reminded me of the last days of my own uncle, Thomas Connally. He was a bachelor who spent most of his life helping other people. Did this man, then, lose his dignity when he was struck with inoperable cancer and could no longer control his life or his giving? Did he lose his dignity through his dependency on doctors, nurses, family, and friends? Was he "degraded" when he finally had to receive hospice care from us? Did he lose his dignity when friends fed him ice cream or chopped ice, when they eased his sufferings with medication? Did he lose his dignity when he had to be turned or washed?

My uncle was a proper and private man. Of course he was embarrassed at times; he also likely worried that he was imposing on us. What he found out in the last weeks of his life, however, was more than he had known through all the earlier years: He was loved and worthy of love, even in the simple and frightening truth of human weakness. He also gave us the opportunity to express our love for him—to give to him, even to hold his hand, as we had never done before.

To die with dignity does not mean to die without anguish or terrible dependency on others. Dignity is a function of personhood. To die with dignity is to die in fidelity to one's personal endowment. The challenge for others is to recognize and respect such dignity.

Television talk shows are now frequented by guests who want to die because they are overweight, desperately in need of a sex change, or depressed because they cannot have the lover they desire. The reality that these distressed people fail to see is that their *estimation* of their value is not the same as their actual value. Our estimation of our worth or dignity is notoriously influenced by cultural and interpersonal standards of approval, attractiveness, and success. A person without a job or with confused sexual identity may feel worthless, but that is not a justification for suicide. It is an indication of pathology.

Physical pathologies and the suffering they can bring are a different matter, however. Among our most harrowing fears is that of a long and lingering death, years of mindlessness and dependency, premature senility, and nursing home existence. These situations undoubtedly are terrible sacrifices in the name of the life given us, even when physical pain can be alleviated. They are one, however, with any personal anguish inevitably invited—not only when we refuse to kill an aggressor or abort an unwanted child but also when we allow ourselves to love and hold ourselves to truth. The issue of our moral life is not an issue of enhancing pleasure or ensuring ease. It is an issue of fidelity to who and what we are.

Derek Humphry, who believes that "everyone has a right to suicide," has written a bestselling "how-to" book called *Final Exit*.[28] Humphry's manual is bereft of any question concerning intrinsic human dignity, although he often mentions death with dignity. He celebrates the "free" choice of those who might wish to terminate their lives, but he presumes a pristine freedom wherein men and women have somehow decided that they have no longer a reason to live.

How great is a freedom, however, if people are continuously programmed to believe that life in itself is not worth living in the first place? How "free," for example, was Humphry's wife Ann (who, with Humphry, helped her own parents die) when she committed suicide in 1991 after finding out that she had breast cancer and her husband left her? Why would she allege in her suicide note that Humphry had impeded her recovery and induced her despair? "There. You got what you wanted. Ever since I was diagnosed as having cancer you have done everything conceivable to precipitate my death. . . . You will have to live with this until you die. May you never, ever forget." The Humphrys had "assisted" Ann's parents in their double suicide five years earlier under conditions that Ann came to believe were close to murder. She also claimed that Humphry actually suffocated his first wife in her "assisted" death. On October 14, 1991, Derek Humphry "took out a half-page advertisement in the *New York Times* that, to the casual reader, might have seemed like a heartfelt eulogy to his former wife. 'Sadly, for much of her life Ann was dogged by emotional problems, and . . . her life was a series of peaks and troughs,' the ad said. . . . Asked why he had placed the ad, Humphry said flatly: 'Damage control.'"[29]

The point of this story is not *ad hominem*. It is to suggest how complex our motives are, whether we think we must "help" another die or seek help to die ourselves. In our culture, the notion of "death with dignity" often is framed in terms of the extrinsic values held by the people around us or society at large. In such a context, many terminally ill people clearly may feel coerced to die because of subtle psychological, social, or economic pressures.

The Black Stork was a film shown commercially in U.S. movie theaters from 1916 to the early 1920s that became something of a cult piece until 1940. It may have lost its appeal because of the ascendency of genocide and euthanasia in Germany. *The Black Stork* was part of the racial purification movement that captured imaginations not only in Europe but in the United States. As Martin Pernick recounts in his book, *The Black Stork*, in an 1898 treatise titled "Degeneracy" a dental surgeon and medical professor proposed selective infanticide. In 1900, Dr. William D. McKim recommended the killing of "institutionally hereditary defectives," among whom he included the retarded, alcoholics, and burglars. Famous psychologist Stanley Hall wanted no medical treatment for "moribund sick, defectives and criminals, because by aiding them to survive it interferes with the process of wholesome natural selection." In 1906, Dr. G. Frank Lydston called for sterilizing the unfit and gassing to death the "driveling imbecile." These accounts are only part of the background of the film, which is the subject of Pernick's harrowing treatment of eugenics and the death of defectives in American medicine.[30] Instructively, Pernick's book ends with observations on the damaged human lives terminated by Dr. Jack Kevorkian.

Kevorkian, a pathologist who has brought the utilitarian principle to its full rationalization, still shocks the public with the simplicity of his logic. He has suggested that capital criminals or others who request suicide ought to be harvested for organs while they are still alive so that some good use might come from their death. Kevorkian insists that he is at the service of freedom. Yet how "free" is the person who wants to end his or her life? If I can sell my organs to help my family, am I free?[31] If I can get out of their way and not cause them discomfort, am I free in deciding to do so? If I am poor and can sell my organs to make an easy life for those I love, am I "free" in that consideration? Am I "free" if I am considered degenerate by my culture? Even the most obvious pressures of the market are unquestioned by Kevorkian's apologists.[32]

Aligned with this misleading and utopian notion of autonomy, the complementary tactic of dehumanization increases the likelihood that more humans become candidates for beneficent killing. Robert J. Lifton portrayed this nightmarish tendency well: "If, at the heart of one's professional identity, one becomes easily susceptible to the idea that mental patients—and possibly other groups as well—lack ordinary human qualities, and hence to the idea of eliminating that group in favor of the ostensible health of all others, one might also be amenable to embracing a new therapy . . . the large Nazi vision of curing by killing."[33] Lifton's work was subtitled "Medical Killing and the Psychology of Genocide."

The crux in all euthanasia issues is the intent to terminate a human life. The purpose may be to alleviate pain; the motive might be compassion for someone living in misery. The intent to kill, however, in each case carries with it a deeper wound than those borne in our bodies. It is a cutting into the heart of ethics itself—an admission that human vulnerability, our very condition as embodied, is degraded and undignified. The response of an individual or a community that values the intrinsic dignity of persons, however, is not to kill the sufferer or eliminate the wounded but to alleviate the suffering and affirm the sufferer's goodness, regardless of the deprivation, the loss, or the presumed shame of human frailty. There is no doubt that a dying person's suffering and death need not be prolonged or that invasive and extraordinary procedures need not be pursued. What is required of us is to live and act in a way that entails acknowledging that no pain or dying or "degenerate" condition robs us of our intrinsic dignity. The direct choice to kill damaged persons betrays that truth.[34]

8

Reviving Personal Life

When do you feel most yourself? (This is different from the question of when you feel more of *a* self, also from the question of when you feel most *alive*.) The answer will not be exactly the same as when you feel most real. People feel most themselves when they are "in contact" with parts of themselves usually not saliently present in their consciousness, dwelling in unaccustomed emotions, integrating these into closer connection with the more familiar portions of themselves. In thoughtful walks in the woods, contemplating the ocean, meditation, or intimate conversations with a friend, deeper parts of oneself are brought into awareness and integrated with the rest, producing a greater serenity of self, a sense of a more substantial self.

Robert Nozick [1]

"It's just the same story a doctor once told me," observed the elder. "He was a man getting on in years, and undoubtedly clever. . . . 'I love humanity,' he said, 'but I wonder at myself. The more I love humanity in general, the less I love man in particular. In my dreams,' he said, 'I often make plans for the service of humanity. . . . Yet I am incapable of living in the same room with anyone for two days together. I know from experience. As soon as anyone is near me, his personality disturbs me and restricts my freedom. . . . I become hostile to people the moment they come close to me. But it has always happened that the more I hate men individually the more I love humanity.'"

Fyodor Dostoyevsky [2]

Money, the word descended from the name of a Roman Goddess in whose sacred temple gold coins were made, infiltrates the psyche as no other human invention. Money can inspire the most euphoric and transitory pleasures and the most suicidal depression. . . . Totemic in the extreme, the "almighty dollar," can encompass and symbolize love,

138

self-esteem, freedom, power, security, dependency, separateness, strength, weakness, goodness, and evil. That money is quantifiable and amenable to accumulation causes it to be lined up against much that is less measurable in life. It becomes a stand-in for the relative intimacy between two people, and, decades after the fact, it is still capable of representing all the undelivered nonfinancial affection someone craved as a child. During a break-up or divorce money regularly represents the absence of love and an advanced weapon of revenge.

Donald Katz [3]

Has it [the world] terrors, they are our terrors; has it abysses, those abysses belong to us; are dangers at hand, we must try to love them.

Rainer Maria Rilke[4]

THE CHOICE OF REALITIES

"When do I feel most myself?" Philosopher Robert Nozick warns us that the answer is not necessarily the same as when we feel like "a" self or even "most alive," not even when we feel most "real." Could this be because the "self" we construct is shaped by hidden codes of "aliveness" and "reality" that somehow are not at the core of our being as persons? "Reality" often serves as a rebuke to what we know is truest, deepest, and dearest in us. "Face the facts," "get real," "be realistic," "lighten up and accept the world" are proffered as the bottom line of life.

What determines the "real," however? Who has dictated and constructed the "reality" we presume in the dogmatic propositions of "the real world"? "Look out for Number One." "It's a dog-eat-dog world." "Everybody is getting a little on the side." "Looking good is everything." These are firmly held beliefs of the dominant "reality system" in the culture around us. Our choice is either to accept them or be doomed as unrealistic, utopian, idealistic.

This book focuses on the foundation of ethics, wherein the moral world is grounded in the reality of human personhood. The fact that we are persons is why we experience the world ethically, why we inevitably feel moral outrage and make judgments about value—even though we might not be able to justify or rationalize our outrage. I argue that if we are going to take morality seriously, we must know what being a human person means, who counts as a person, and what the implications of personhood are. Chapter 7 applied these foundations to a range of issues that touch on the most basic arena of human action: the killing of human beings. Rather than address an array of concrete issues, I offer one foundational principle for a life committed to a radically personalist ethics. For many readers, however, this principle will seem wholly "unrealistic." How can one ever expect anyone to accept a moral principle never to intend to kill a human being?

I choose not to argue extensively through particular cases or applications for three reasons. First, I think that our moral positions rarely are changed through argument. Argument is only a part of rationality and rationality only one part of experience. The other parts, often neglected, also must be addressed. Even in the case of the general ethical theory I have offered, I have done so more with the hope that I could provide philosophical justification for men and women who intuitively are committed to the dignity of persons than with a confidence that I could easily change minds.

A second reason that argument over cases is rarely profitable is that, if we are honest, we realize that in practice, we often are unable or unwilling to make the very choices that we know are best theoretically. A theoretical truth cannot compete with a lived crisis.

My final reason is the "reality" problem.[5]

A person or a group of people can be so deeply formed by a "reality system" that depersonalizes them that even the most simple themes of personalism—fidelity, intrinsic value, commitment, ascetical simplicity, promise-keeping—simply do not make sense. Specific practices of personal virtue can seem outlandish. Rather than seriously consider a way of life that is not based upon killing in self-defense, retaliation, or the exercise of force over others, we "accept the real world" by arming ourselves or our nation against all enemies. Rather than consider the possibility that physician-assisted suicide and abortion might be profound rejections of our humanity, we invoke the right to determine our lives without examining the implications of what we are determined to do. Rather than engage the persons around us in family or civic communion, we learn to sit passively before a television set; we learn not to sit on our front porches; we learn to fear the young and the stranger; we expect nightly violence. Accommodations—seclusion or security—are made. It's the "real" world.

Thus, we capitulate to depersonalization. When we disengage ourselves from the personal realm, we suffer a failure of recollection that our lives can be empowered by both solitude and solidarity. We forget that communities can engage and empower us, as they have done in the great civil rights movements of the past, in labor organizations, and in political resistance to unjust authority. We fail to understand that concerted national effort can engage and even change the expectations and behavior of a populace.

In the contexts of cultural formation and the effective change of human behavior, we may be startled to remember that as recently as the 1960s, every elevator in every building of every town had ash trays outside them. Automobiles usually had four or five. All tables at restaurants had them. Waiting rooms, doctors' offices, conference tables had three or four. Many movie theaters had ash trays attached to the backs of seats. Airplanes had them snuggled into the arm rests.

That situation has all changed—so much so that smokers may well be the only class of individuals whom we roundly condemn. When I asked an eager, intelligent student (a "relativist," she called herself) if there were *any* behavior that she might think intrinsically disordered or morally wrong, she said with a quizzical expression, "Smoking and cruelty to animals?" No student could have *imagined* such a response four decades ago. Perceived "reality" systems change—sometimes for the good, sometimes not.

Culture "cultivates" us with formation. As such, it dominates the "formation" and content of our moral judgments. The only basis for the judgments we make is the information we have received. Students hate to hear this. So do teachers—even those who celebrate the influences of culture. For if we acknowledge that our judgments about reality are profoundly influenced by the programming of our culture, we must at least be willing to question that culture. We must at least be open to other modes of experience than those that are culturally reinforced. Culture provides the construction of reality that most of us apply to our ethical judgment. If culture inculcates attitudes of unfettered choice, low tolerance of pain, high approval for appearance and performance, it will foster consciences that are prone to depersonalizing choices. Hence most attempts at providing ethical arguments in the abstract will fail—if not in the attempt, surely in the moment of choice.

Consequently, I devote the first part of this chapter to a description of our "reality system," especially in contemporary North America (though friends in Africa, Europe, Australia, and Central America have said the characterization applies to them as well). This "reality system" is

inextricably related to every aspect of life. A consuming, capitalist culture places a tremendous priority on our relation to produced, purchased,
and accumulated objects, rather than persons. Our self-understanding as
well as our relationship to others is mediated through consumer consciousness and its values of possession, quantity, control, appearance,
and function. Thus, as *Worth* magazine suggests in one of the quotations
at the beginning of this chapter, money serves as an immensely powerful
criterion for worth, value, and happiness. Money, in conjunction with
the objects and the satisfactions it promises, is a "reality" principle that
overrides the most intimate and universal values we may hold. Totemic
and almighty, it encompasses identity, relationship, freedom, goodness,
and evil. "Money can inspire the most euphoric and transitory pleasures
and the most suicidal depression." This is the ethos, even the spirituality,
of capitalism—not as the celebrated means of economic ingenuity and
private enterprise but as a habit of being, a way of life.[6]

The second and more important goal of this chapter is to suggest
patterns of living that provide an alternative information system: the
formation of personal habits of being. A commitment to a life of ethical
personalism, an understanding of its "reality," can only be discovered in
the lived reality, the "habitus," of personal existence. In solitude before
the immensity of nature or the depth of our interior aspirations, in the
joys and crucibles of committed relationship, in the discovery of dignity
in the most vulnerable and broken of persons, we break through to the
indubitable "realness" of the personal realm.

A "habitus" of personal existence, a manner of living in which the
virtues or "strengths" of personal life are exercised, empowers us to
become the kind of humans who will be personally authentic in our
moral choices and faithful to the reality of what we are.[7] People who
have tasted the truth of what being a unique and irreplaceable person
means—whether discovered in the citadel of solitude, the aura of profound relationship, or a liberating encounter with culturally and philo-
sophically "marginal" humans—will not only be less inclined to succumb
to the blandishments of capitalism. They will also be less inclined to kill.

THE "REALITY" OF CONSUMER CAPITALISM

The "real world" of contemporary American life is not an expression of personal existence. It is the expression, instead, of a media fan-

tasy that celebrates the marvelous magic of money and possession as
foundational goods. They make us feel more alive, secure, and important. They give us value, substance, and visibility. They signal
importance and dominance. They bestow a transcendent value on the
possessor. They determine the future of our lives and relationships, the
stability of our institutions, the solvency of our academic departments,
the success of our careers.

James Twitchell's *Lead Us Into Temptation: The Triumph of American Materialism* is an often-humorous rejoinder to the foregoing concerns. It is
not so much a refutation of the thesis that consumer capitalism has diminished personal life as a hymn to capitalism's success, albeit at a price.
The cost is the consumption of our own interior lives, of our relationships and of our sense of human solidarity. Although Twitchell insists
that we have grown stronger by believing in what he calls the "ridicu-
lous myths" surrounding the possession of commodities, although com-
merce has become the central "register of selfhood," although style and
packaging have replaced substance, Twitchell announces a strange new
world of "freedom":

> Consumerism is wasteful, it is devoid of otherworldly concerns, it lives
> for today and celebrates the body. It overindulges and spoils the young
> with impossible promises. It encourages recklessness, living beyond one's
> means, gambling. Consumer culture is always new, always without a past.
> Like religion, which it has displaced, it afflicts the comfortable and
> comforts the afflicted. It is heedless of the truly poor who cannot gain
> access to the loop of meaningful information that is carried through its
> ceaseless exchanges. It is a one-dimensional world, a wafer-thin world, a
> world low on significance and high on glitz, a world without yesterdays.
>
> Getting and spending has been the most passionate, and often the
> most imaginative endeavor of modern life. We have done more than
> acknowledge that the good life starts with material life, as the ancients
> did. We have made stuff the dominant prerequisite of organized society.
> Things "R" Us. Consumption has become production. While this is
> dreary and depressing to some, as doubtless it should be, it is liberating
> and democratic to many more.[8]

Capitalism assuredly is not the *only* force of depersonalization in
the world; totally administered states, religions, ideologies, and cults all
pose as unquestioned "realities" before which every impulse of personal
existence must bow. Yet Twitchell unknowingly unmasks the systemic

power of a system that promises freedom but delivers a one-dimensional, paper-thin world of producing and accumulating objects as the meaning and goal of human life.

In the case of American capitalism, the immediacy and power of its "reality" is felt in a range of experiences: making a killing on the stock market, shopping at a mall, dreaming of the winning lottery ticket, winning admiration for our appearance or achievement, or partaking in the liturgies of rock concerts. When such things happen, we feel like somebody. We have value. We sense that we are connected and confirmed. We feel transcendence as well.

The fabulously popular rock band U2 ended its early 1990s concerts with the message, "Thank you for shopping at Zoo TV." This remark was preeminently appropriate. Although U2 was a commercial success—drawing $30 from 40,000 fans at each venue—the band's tour was a high-tech, postmodern critique of consumerism as a propaganda and formation system. Bono, the Edge, Adam Clayton, and Larry Mullen had moved away from their straightforward, urgent seriousness into a highly politicized but ironic style. The dimensions of the techno-consumer world had become so vast, they could dwarf and domesticate even the countercultural pretensions of a rock band. The band's new strategy was an "in-your-face" mockery of media and market forces. Yet Bono was deadly serious in his interpretation of contemporary culture. In a *Rolling Stone* interview, unmasked of irony, he complained:

> I don't think religion has anything to do with God anymore or very rarely has. It is also becoming clear that the material world is not enough for anybody. We had a century of being told by the intelligentsia that we're two-dimensional creatures, that if something can't be proved, it can't exist. That's over now. Transcendence is what everybody, in the end, is on their knees for, running at speed toward, scratching at, kicking at. That's why music is, for me, important.[9]

The hunger for "transcendence" is not lost on the consumer culture and the world of advertising. In fact, much of the kneeling, running, and searching in America is still intently focused on the production, purchasing, and possessing of objects that are mystically endowed with promises that only a personal relationship or religious system can deliver.

In a 1989 article in the *Journal of Consumer Research*, Belk, Wallendorf, and Sherry noted that shopping represents much more than the satisfaction of everyday material needs. "Consumption can become a vehicle of transcendent experience: That is, consumer behavior exhibits certain aspects of the sacred." Like religion, commodities can convey a belief "in something significantly more powerful and extraordinary than the self—a need to transcend existence as a mere biological being coping with the everyday world."[10]

Some companies that manufacture our most "real" identity tags serve as our moral and psychological advisors as well. Benetton, which chose a rainbow of condoms as a symbol of its "United Colors" theme, has marketed its clothes under the guise of compassion with pictures of bombed-out villages, dead soldiers, and AIDS sufferers. Conscience and social awareness have become something to wear as a fashion statement.

Nike Corporation, principal in the school of social conditioning, announces the cultural curriculum over its loudspeakers: "This is your life. And there are no rules. And there are no grades." But there are rules, and there are grades. The awesome power of commodities dictates how we must look, act, dress, talk, and think. Children will sob for the lack of Adidas. Teens might kill for leather jackets. A nation will go to war against an oil-rich country "to preserve our way of life."[11]

The displacement of persons by purchased objects is the underlying imperative of consumer "reality." "I'm looking for a meaningful relationship, and I've found it at Saks Fifth Avenue." Thus a capitalist's advertisement baldly confirms Marx's claim that the commodity world has a strange religious quality wherein men and women relate to things as if the things were persons (material relations become social relations), and they relate to persons as if the persons were objects (social relations are transformed into material relations). Marx gave this phenomenon the now famous name of "the commodity fetish."

> There is a definite social relation between men that assumes, in their eyes, the fantastic form of a relation between things. In order, therefore, to find an analogy, we must have recourse to the mist-enveloped regions of the religious world. In that world the productions of the human brain appear as independent beings endowed with life, and entering in to relations both with one another and the human race. So it is in the world of commodities with the products of men's hands. This I call the Fetishism which attaches itself to the products of labor, so soon as they are produced as commodities.[12]

If consumer products are sacral fetishes, the mall is the cathedral of consumption, where we process to ease our hunger for relationship and transcendence. We purchase products called Absolut, Eternity, Infiniti, Opium, Love, Idole, Happiness, Joy.

In an ultimate "reality" and value system, its disciples become like the absolute they follow. In the commercial god, the true believers find themselves recreated. They are now made not in the image and likeness of a personal reality but after the fashion of a commodity. This is the metaphysics, the anthropology, the ethic, the spirituality of consumerism.

The "habitus" of capitalism is a mode of life in which human existence is ontologically grounded in the world of things. In such a world, conceiving of persons as objects, instruments, or possessions is no difficult leap. Yet understanding one's life as having any intrinsic worth or value apart from the externals of appearance, utility, and productivity is quite difficult. We learn to feel "real" not in intimacy or solitude or human solidarity but in the act of buying up and relating to objects. Moreover, because we can control our relationships to objects much better than we can control our relationships to persons, the personal realm is reduced to a lesser, more threatening, value.

The dehumanized world evoked by Bono and U2—a performance band dwarfed by a huge stage, outsized by deafening sounds of amplification and massive screened messages, diminished by countless advertisements—has been encountered before. Orwell's *1984* and the Nazis' Nuremberg rallies were forerunners of U2's "Zoo TV": They constructed rituals and extravaganzas in which men and women were shrunk by images of Moloch, seduced by ersatz religious feeling, and swept into an illusion of solidarity. Bono and his band recreate the experience as an embodiment of America's consumer and media culture, where the abiding human hunger for fulfillment and transcendence is channeled, as Bono suggests, into hawking and hunting for merchandise. Yet as the song at the end of U2's concert (while dazzling lights flash "Thank you for shopping at Zoo TV") goes, "I still haven't found what I'm looking for."[13]

REVIVING PERSONAL SOLITUDE

We are looking for the truth, not images, of ourselves and our world, for only the truth is the grounds for love. We cannot love what we do not know. We cannot experience being loved if we do not experience ourselves being known. We cannot even love ourselves—as Nozick and Dostoievsky suggest—if we do not face and accept the truth of what we are.

The recovery of moral consciousness requires the recovery of lived personal existence. We cannot begin to disengage from the "reality" system of products and money unless we experience personal reality in the habits of our life. Jacob Needleman has wisely observed that the actual moral failure of our culture is not our marketing of value and truth; it is the fact that buying and selling have become our most intense and vivid experiences. The direct experiences of personal love and commitment have faded. "If a person marries for money rather than love or duty, it is not necessarily because he prefers money to love or duty, but because he has not experienced the real force of love or duty."[14]

To make the personal world "vivid and intense," we must undertake a recovery of practices and habits that dispose us to experience ourselves and the world in a personal manner. This "practicing" of the personal virtues is more strategic in the formation of an "ethical life" and the execution of moral choice than any argument or exhortation.

This practice first requires the "meditative" habit of personal solitude. Disengagement and withdrawal from the "givenness" of daily life has been a recurring theme of the history of philosophy—not as a rejection of the external world or interpersonal relationships but as a focusing on the internal aspects of experience. Thus, Marcus Aurelius and Descartes offered "Meditations," Pascal his *Pensées*; Augustine his *Confessions*, Aquinas his poetry, Russell and Sartre their autobiographies. Thoreau had his *Walden*:

> I went to the woods because I wished to live deliberately, to confront only the essential fact of life, and see if I could not learn what it had to teach, and not, when I came to die, discover that I had not lived. I did not wish to live what was not life, living is so dear.[15]

Solitude generates the unsettling question of what we might be when we are not producing, performing, or consuming. Appearances, comparisons, and achievements mean little in true solitude. How we look will change. What we have produced can be replaced. The ways we have surpassed others will be yet surpassed. Solitude poses the possibility that we bring something to this world that is preeminently "our own," unique to us, not merely a function of performance and comparative achievement or any other "mirroring" of culture and competition.

Undeniably, if solitude is taken as some anchor or "starting point" that grounds all other arenas of our experience, it can lead to a disengaged and solipsistic view of our being. It need not, however. Augustine was an accomplished politician, Aquinas a prolific writer and courageous ground-breaker in the bridging of cultures, Pascal a scientist and polemicist, Thoreau an activist in civil disobedience, and the reclusive Descartes an inexhaustible letter writer. Solitude enables us to contact what and who we are when we are not acting or performing or collecting.

The discovery of our own personal citadels need not lead us into isolated atomic cocoons that are disconnected from our social world. When we meet ourselves in solitude, we are forced to face the vulnerability of our personal being. Although true solitude demands a stripping away of the external pretenses and roles we project to justify and legitimate ourselves, in the moment of our ontological nakedness we discover not an "autonomous self" but a chastened and vulnerable ego whose existence itself is gift and whose actuality is given only by the context of history and culture. The truth of our embodied personhood is the truth of our radical contingency and limitation. We avoid this truth in the flight from aloneness.[16] We are not beings in control of our existence or our value. We receive it. We embrace it. We do not construct it. We repress this truth when we refuse to accept the limits of our embodied existence and the constraints of our moral consciousness. The truths we avoid in our illusions of domination, control, and limitlessness are the same truths we embrace in solitude: We are creatures. We are contingent. We die.

Tolstoy's Ivan Ilyich is the perfect exemplar of our fear of death. He can understand the death of others, but not his own. In unguarded moments, however, the thought of it is inescapable:

> He could not understand it; and he endeavored to put away this thought as false, unjust, unwholesome, and to supplant it with other thoughts true and wholesome. But this thought, not merely as a thought, but, as it were, a reality, kept recurring and taking form before him.
>
> And he summoned in place of this thought other thoughts, one after the other, in the hope of finding succor in them. He strove to return to his former course of reasoning, which hid from him of old the thought of death.[17]

The terror that can mount when we face our finitude is one with our fear of intimacy and our fear of the visibly wounded who no longer have pretenses of control or performance. It also is one with the philosophical avoidance of mortality and the political posturing of enduring power. In solitude, once the applause has stopped, the distractions quieted, and the plans let go, the upsetting thought may occur: I *am* no longer if I am no longer in control. I *am* no longer if I am not useful or productive. Such thoughts, of course, are what lead us to think we have no worth or value if we are dependent and helpless.

"An anxious resistance to death largely drives the broader civilizing activities of humankind, whether in the reproduction of the species, the military defense of nations, the pursuit of careers, the aspiration to command and power, the publication of books, the creation of fortunes . . . or the daily jostling for prestige."[18] The thought of our death drives what medical ethicist Daniel Callahan calls the "troubled dream of life," wherein we cling to illusions of control and mastery. It drives the technology-driven decisions to prolong our dying rather than accept it. It drives our anxieties about helplessness and dependency.[19] In solitude, bereft of distraction, stripped of pretense, unlike Tolstoy's Ilyich, we allow ourselves to experience our creatureliness.

Our animality reminds us of such creaturehood: our needs and neediness, our fragile gestation and birthing and equally frail diminishment and dying, our inability to control our destinies and our bodies at the margins of life. Thus, we might understandably wish to have our being wholly identified with our brains, its higher states, its more elegant and controlled expressions. That is not what we human persons are, however. We are incarnate, fleshly beings. Our brains themselves look like mounds of meat. The shock of our enfleshed condition jolts us, like Ilyich, into self-confrontation. Rather than inducing panic or self-rejection, however, such moments of recognition also beckon us to accept our truth so that we may begin to love ourselves as we are.

Thus, in solitude, we may discover our grace. Being present to our own presence in the world, being present to our bodies in the discipline and habit of quiet, we discover the one reality that we are empowered to give to the world and that cannot be replaced by any other. That reality is our own capacity to become related to our own life story, to take ownership of it and bestow it on others. We are led to realize that the measure of our lives is not what we have built or accumulated but what we have given ourselves to. The very power of our love, the range of our hope, the strength of our faith is found in our fragility. They cannot be a function of control and demand, lest they lose their very meaning. They are incommensurable with quantity, measurement, or comparison, for they are the fruit of our very uniqueness and the ground of all human solidarity. No one is first or better in this realm of personhood, for no one has any other personal life to give but one's own. Without this encountering of our own interior personal existence, our freedom, our responsibility, and our capacity to care will remain little more than mere words or ideology. The philosophical term for such experiences is the reflexively conscious encounter with life.

In solitude, in withdrawal from the noise and clatter of culture, in disengagement from the imperatives to produce, to win, to consume, we allow one dimension of our personal existence to command our attention. Yet this is only *one* dimension of personal life. Its truth must be tested out in the full range of our being as embodied persons, as interpersonal and social. Human solitude and interiority cannot even be what it is without the "other."

RECOVERING PERSONAL RELATIONSHIPS

In the second thematic passage at the beginning of this chapter, Dostoyevsky sets the scene between Madam Hohlakov and the mystic Zossima in *The Brothers Karamazov* in the context of a personal crisis. Madam Hohlakov has gone to old Zossima for advice. She's afraid she is losing her faith, especially her faith in the afterlife. The monk tells her that love, not faith, is the real issue. She immediately agrees: She has a problem with love.

As Zossima points out, however, we experience our personal crises most truly not as isolated interior struggles, not as theoretical issues of love or justice, not even as compassion for the downtrodden who may come to our doors or accost us on the street. At our best, we can manage distant strangers with a smile, especially if the encounter is not too long and there are not too many "follow-up" expectations. The existential problem is the person I must live and labor with: the person at hand; the person in my community, my family, my circle of friends. One can entertain the largest dreams in the stillness of solitude. One can theoretically aspire to the heights of fairness and equity. In relationship, however, all is tested. In the presence of the other, I am faced, I am named, I am called forth into relationship. This relationship, however, demands a recognition of another person as more than a function of my own ego or desires.

Zossima recounts the story of a humanitarian but cynical doctor who harbored great dreams of justice and service but could not stand the "restriction" on his freedom that any other person presents. His "humanitarianism" crashes on the reality of human relationship. He becomes hostile the moment people come close. When Madame Hohlakov recognizes herself in Zossima's story, she is initially crushed. The old monk insists, however, that her journey in faith and love is finally begun. She has accepted the truth.

> Avoid being scornful, both to others and to yourself. What seems to you bad within will grow purer from the very fact of your observing it in yourself. Avoid fear, too, though fear is only the result of falsehood. Never be frightened at your own faint-heartedness in attaining love. Don't be too frightened even at your evil actions. I am sorry I can say nothing more consoling to you, for love in action is a harsh and dreadful thing compared with love in dreams. Love in dreams is greedy for immediate action, rapidly performed and in the sight of all. Men will even give their lives if only the ordeal does not last long but is soon over, with all looking on and applauding as though on the stage. But active love is labor and fortitude, and for some people too, a complete science.[20]

Moral ideals—especially the ideal of love—are tested not in argument but in the "harsh and dreadful love" required in our daily struggles with each other. There is a spirituality of politics. There is a politics in our personal relationships. The pathologies of the social order, whether spawned in fear or falsehood, are mirrored in our own private disorders.

Asking governments to lay down their arms is one thing. Disarming ourselves before the enemy with a neighbor's face is quite another. Some of our contemporary "moral saints" confirm this distinction. Jean Vanier, founder of the l'Arche communities, observes that our love for the "handicapped" sometimes seems so much easier than the love we are called to give our "nonhandicapped" collaborators. Mother Teresa admitted that greater asceticism is demanded of us by community than by the most spartan dress and the plainest foods. Dorothy Day's journals are more filled with self-critique, especially of her relations with people, than with critiques of society.[21]

Personal relationships test all theories, whether they are social, spiritual, or psychological. Community and intimacy are unions of persons at greater closeness and intensity than connections of nation, class, or convenience. Such unions are relationships of intimacy (*intime*)—relationships in depth. Thus, true friendship, close solidarity, lasting commitments, and covenanted family are opportunities for profound experiences of community. Our moral sensibility and passion are forged in our relations of committed intimacy—in which we are unmasked, in which we are known and loved for who we are, in which our pretenses are displayed and our vulnerability is laid open.

Only in those places where we are known in depth, *intime*, can we be loved in truth. There too, however, we can be most deeply hurt. Naturally, then, we experience powerful aversions to intimacy, relationship, and community. We are tempted to hold ourselves in, to protect ourselves with impregnable defenses, to assure our personal security. We entertain the illusion that if we protect ourselves from being known, we will never be vulnerable, unguarded, and open to attack. Thus, we reproduce in our communities and families the very patterns of defense and aggression, injustice and denial, that rules the age and the rulers of the age.

Yet if we enter the truth of relationship, if we live in community, we must be willing to face our egoisms and fears; we must be willing to take off the armor of isolation and toughness. We may indeed be shamed, like Madame Hohlakov, before the gaze of someone who knows us, but we also will experience the power of our truth. We will discover what being loved for who and what we are means. We need not—because we cannot—"fake it" through life. Though often vulnerable, broken, and morally flawed, we can experience being vigorously graced with our own irreplaceable gift of love that we are allowed to bestow on each other.

Authentic community, to be sure, is a rare phenomenon in contemporary culture, where relationship and intimacy seem to be so assiduously avoided. Most of our energies are directed to behaviors that lead us away from relationship. Competition inhabits our work, homes, and schools. Hidden and unquestioned imperatives that we must earn more but care less are part of our cultural myth. Even the professionalism of "caregivers" can serve as a disengagement from caring.

In a 1993 broadcast of "The Health Quarterly" by the Public Broadcasting System, one of the topics was the phenomenon of euthanasia in Holland. In one case, we see a man afflicted with AIDS who wishes to die. The physician displays a discomfort that is clearly readable by the man who is choosing death. The man asks his doctor, "Is this difficult for you?" "No," the doctor replies, "I've had three others." The caregiver refuses to communicate or even acknowledge his care for the patient before him, even though in discussions with other physicians he admits that his greatest stress is in controlling his feelings. A second case involves a retired professor who seemingly has the early stages of Alzheimer's disease. He is asked whether he wants to die. "No," he says, "but I see no reason to go on living." Watching these cases is excruciating: In the first instance, the doctor cannot even bring himself to admit that assisting in the suicide is personally painful for him, and in the second instance, no friends or professionals will tell the old man that it might mean a difference to *them* if he would choose to live.[22] The two patients are studies in depression and hunger for anyone who might *care* that they keep living; the distanced professionals seem incapable of giving it, however. Such is the harrowing reality of authentic relationship and human solidarity.

Our media rarely present any images of men and women who are capable of enduring commitment or personal intimacy other than random sexual encounter. Civic virtues, friendship, personal care, and neighborliness seem almost utopian qualities of a distant past. We may even feel at times that community is an illusion, that commitment is an impossibility, that covenant is a dream of another world.

The lives we build together in friendship, community, or family are much more than personal needs or interpersonal comforts. They are strategic choices we make as social and political beings—not only to test the reality of our commitment to justice or the genuineness of our "spiritual" lives but as leaven in a culture that is desperately in need of human community.

Philosophers of "otherness" and "intersubjectivity"—from Aristotle on "Friendship" to John Macmurray and Martin Buber—have investigated the constitution of our personal existence through mutuality.[23] The most confirming data, however, always come from the experience of relationship.

REVEALING HUMAN VULNERABILITY

Behind every moral failure is a denial of the truth of what we are. This denial is a repression of our personal reality and a denial of creatureliness. The problem is compounded by our refusal to *accept* our moral failure. Just as solitude is an exercise in unmasking pretense, just as committed relationships demand a relinquishment of social disguise, a willingness to encounter the vulnerabilities of our social and political world will evoke our compassion for the wounded of our world as well as our own existence. It also will expose our fear—not only of the undeniably wounded but of the deniable wound within us.

The "habit" of personal being I propose is the practice of exposing ourselves to data that can be provided only by men and women for whom "the American Dream" might be a nightmare. These people are the unproductive, the undesirable, the undeserving, the unwanted.

Many of us in this culture are bereft of any first-hand experience of people who are considered worthless in terms of external values. In the absence of such experience, believing such people are expendable or better off dead than alive is easy for us. This attitude occurs in the depersonalization of criminals, the demonization of the "enemy," and the degradation of entire classes of persons who do not "count" as wanted, successful, or fully functioning. The poor become abstractions, rather than living reminders of our shared human condition. Other races become caricatures, rather than peoples who might complement our own gifts and challenge our perspectives. Terminally ill persons are "vegetative" nightmares of dependency and distaste, rather than brothers or sisters who reveal our ultimate vulnerability. Perhaps that is why the only way we can deal with the reality of damaged humans and the rebuke they profer to our illusions of autonomy and control is to theoretically remove them from our vaunted "community of persons."

The rare writer or uncommon television program reminds us of a greater truth. Oliver Sacks' riveting tales of profoundly damaged persons are charged with a love and admiration for the very people whom we presume would be better off dead than alive.[24] Robert Coles' accounts of the poor and disenfranchised, who might be considered productive and managerial failures, give a range and depth to his psychiatric writings and teaching of medical students at Harvard.[25] Elie Wiesel and Viktor Frankl display a range, depth, and passion that was forged in the most horrible crucibles of human vulnerability and evil in concentration camps.[26] Jean-Dominique Bauby, the former editor of *Paris Elle*, dictates *The Diving Bell and the Butterfly* with his one winking eye, revealing the "monstrous, iniquitous" condition of being paralyzed, yet loved and loving, albeit as a shadow of what he was.[27]

We must ask *ourselves*—whether student, philosopher, or citizen—how the experience of the marginal, the wounded, the dying, might lead us to love them, rather than to fear or destroy them.

Mev Puleo was one of the most vibrant and intelligent students I have ever encountered. She loved philosophy, literature, and especially the arts. Her experience of marginal persons in our world—especially those excluded from our American capitalist dream—unleashed her greatest creativity and insight as a photojournalist. In an observation written five years before her death from a brain tumor at the age of 32, she commented,

> Many of us are tempted to be intolerant of the ambiguity and intimidated by the risks of photography and other art forms. Ultimately, I believe we are most daunted by the mystery, the question, the possibility: "It could be us." Through my own photography I strive to bridge the distant worlds of our small globe. I contemplate the mystery. It is us.[28]

Only by entering the life of "those who had not dignity" did she realize that dignity was not a function of performance but of being a human person. For in her own dying, she definitively knew and taught all those around her that the poor "could be us." All of her splendid gifts of word and physical grace relinquished, she became the poor she so deeply wanted to identify with. Bereft of performance and achievement, she was left only with her love and her power to evoke it from us. The truest artists, scientists, philosophers, and businesspeople do not deny human vulnerability but enter it.

Two physicians who also are academicians reveal the same reality. Sheila Cassidy, who has written *Light from the Dark Valley*, recounts her transition from professionalism to the care of "degenerate life":

> It is difficult to explain the love-hate relationships we have with those spectres at the feast of life, gaunt figures with their tissues and their vomit bowls, oblivious to the appalling stench from their foul necrotic tumors. We are not immune to the smell of decaying flesh, and, like anyone, we long to escape to where the air is pure. And yet, cohabiting peacefully with our distaste, is a real love for these broken people. People mutter . . . "How awful! If it were a dog, you'd have it put down." But then, [the patient] is not a dog, but a man with cancer in his mouth, who is living out his last precarious days, loved and cherished in a way that he has never known before. It is in this lavishing of love on patients that the hospice movement

stands in a prophetic relationship to society at large, for it affirms the value of the brain-damaged, the mutilated and the old to a world which values the clever, the physically beautiful and the athletic.[29]

The love-hate quality of our relationships is poignantly true. The good is there to be seen and affirmed, which is love. The guise of the broken body reminds us of the shame we have of our own bodies—woundable, subject to infirmity, powerless before time. That reminder is capable of generating the most profound of hates and fears.[30]

Danielle Darriet received her doctorate in medical science from the University of Bordeaux and pursued specialties in biochemistry and memory; she did research in radiation sciences at the Washington University School of Medicine in the United States before returning to France and the Laboratoire de Psychophysiologie in Talence. After seven years, she resigned her position to become the primary care physician for severely head-injured patients in Berck, France. She reports:

> I am in charge of thirty brain-damaged patients. I have always been fascinated by the brain. It is amazing to see how a brain lesion can alter the behavior of a person. But, as a handicapped woman said, "This body is the envelope, do not stop with looking at the outside; read the letter inside." Five of the patients are in a vegetative state and we can find no way to open the envelope and yet, there is someone there. Five of them are in a low awareness state. For these ten patients, the great suffering is for the family. How can we deal with their affliction? And I wonder, "What is the meaning of this kind of life?" Some of the patients are still dependent but try to communicate whether with language or signs. . . . Finally the others begin to regain independence and their cognitive impairments are really striking. It is terribly difficult to deal with the disturbing and painful symptoms of people who have brain damage. But are they not symptoms of the limitations we all share? So, the patients show me who I am.[31]

No academic research can approximate the willingness of the professional to enter into the life of a "marginal" person and see oneself within. Yet that will, that openness, is required if one is to abide in the realm of personhood. Academic musings may facilitate control of one's thought experiments or logical deductions, but they are an escape from the reality of our condition as embodied persons. Within each of us is the helpless child of a nursery and the broken patient in a nursing home.

Although Jean Vanier is a philosopher, most of his work has been devoted to living with and writing about persons who confound most philosophers and frighten many ordinary people. The experience of encountering men and women whom Nietzsche deemed "degenerate life" changed his life. Nietzsche would have had them killed. We ourselves might rather die than be like them.

> I came to visit them. I was embarrassed, not knowing quite how to communicate with people who couldn't talk very well, and wondering, even if they could, what we would talk about. But I was touched by these men. By some word or gesture or through the look in their eyes they seemed to be saying to me, "Do you love me?" At the time, I was teaching philosophy at the University of Toronto, where my students were interested in my intelligence, in what I could teach them so that they could pass their exams. But these men didn't care about what was in my head; they were interested in my person, in my heart and in my capacity to relate.[32]

Philosophers rarely speak of the "margins" of human personhood—rarer, even, than a philosopher writing of luminous solitude; rarer still than a philosopher's treatise on the devastation and ecstasy of love. This rarity, I propose, exemplifies the fact that many philosophers, like all of us, are not at home with the uncontrollable margins of human existence, with life experiences that force us to reconsider the pretense of the "autonomous man," with "marginal" persons who challenge the belief that personal identity is reducible to the effectiveness and resilence of the brain. Vanier discovered that even wounded personhood could move his heart and evoke his love. The one gift that he could uniquely give to the world was the one gift that the world wanted of him.

Perhaps Charles Taylor has gently suggested why:

> Is the naturalist affirmation conditional on a vision of human nature in the fullness of its health and strength? Does it move us to extend help to the irremediably broken, such as the mentally handicapped, those dying without dignity, fetuses with genetic defects? Perhaps one might judge that it doesn't and that this is a point in favor of naturalism; perhaps effort shouldn't be wasted on these unpromising cases. But the careers of Mother Teresa or Jean Vanier seem to point to a different pattern, emerging from a Christian spirituality. I am obviously not neutral in posing these questions. Even though I have refrained (partly out of delicacy, but largely out of lack

of arguments) from answering them, the reader suspects that my hunch lies towards the affirmative, that I do think naturalist humanism defective in these respects.[33]

In the recovery of personal existence, consequently, one final habit of life recommends itself: to expose our hearts and intellects to the "damaged," the "handicapped," the "defective," and the "avoided." They may reveal to us the deepest truths of our being and the inadequacy of all our philosophies. In avoiding the wounded we may well be avoiding the truth. For what is defective in them serves to remind us of the contingency that is one with our frail embodiment as persons. What we lose by ignoring them may be nothing less than the power of our humanity to call forth and bestow love.

The "center" to which a radical personalist returns is not a controlling "autonomous" ego that somehow constitutes itself in isolation from others or the world. Nor could a "personal" center ever consider itself the center of the world. The very *existence* of a personal history is experienced as gift, not something self-created. So also, the *presence of our personal endowments* is only by gift rather than achievement. This is the meaning of their intrinsic quality and our intrinsic dignity. The value of human persons is something we recognize and respond to, not something we construct or confer. Even the way we exercise and realize these endowments is by grace of gift from the other: the gifts of genetic information and environmental sustenance from our earliest moments, the gifts of birth and nutriment, the gifts of earth and culture, the gifts of the parent's face calling out and naming our identities, the gifts of ready languages and supple traditions.

Our return to the center of personal existence requires the most profound humility, for it is a center that can only *be* if it relinquishes its self. We find within a chastened ego, winnowed of the illusion that one can be a self-made man or woman, freshly aware not only of our portentous powers to know and love freely but also of our tendencies to choose the lie and make ourselves gods.

The admission of our moral failure and the acceptance of our fragile truth as persons cost us our illusions. Yet they provide the only grounds on which love can be based and from which a life of personal freedom can be launched. It is the truth of our human personhood.

Dostoievsky's wise Zossima counseled Madam Hohlakov that her problem was not a loss of faith in God. It was a loss of faith in humanity and herself as well. It was triggered by the disillusionment we suffer when we are forced to face the truth of our moral failure. Yet the recognition itself provides the beginning of the return to the heart of personal existence. The journey would be harsh and dreadful, Zossima warned, but it would be true—and it would make possible a life of love.

So it is with the ethical life, as some philosophers know:

> Truth is stronger than falsehood, however cunning; hope will always triumph over despair, however heavily armed; love, with its readiness for self-sacrifice, is a match for hatred, which for all its threatening visage has fear and cowardice at its heart. We can assess this with utter confidence, because the negative is only possible through the positive and depends upon it. How can death overcome life, when it is the mere negative of life? How can evil be other than parasitic upon good?[34]

Notes

NOTES TO CHAPTER 1

1. Thomas Aquinas, *Summa Theologica*, First Part, Question 29, Article 3. Whether one uses the *Summa Theologica* (New York: Benziger, 1947), the multiple volume *Summa Theologiae* set with commentary and Latin facing pages by Blackfriars (New York: McGraw-Hill, 1963), or *Summa Theologiae: A Concise Translation*, ed. Timothy McDermott (Westminster, Md.: Christian Classics, 1989), the normal notation reads "S.T., Ia. xxix, 3."

2. The specific reference is to Richard Rorty. In *Consequences of Pragmatism* (Boston: Beacon Press, 1988), Rorty appears to call for a dismissal of the great Kantian questions of human identity and purpose. Rorty's present position emerged from his influential *Philosophy and the Mirror of Nature* (Princeton, N.J.: Princeton University Press, 1979). His rejection of the notion that humanity is a "natural kind" with an intrinsic nature endowed with natural powers is developed in *Contingency, Irony and Solidarity* (New York: Cambridge University Press, 1989), wherein any attempt to question where the mysterious phenomena of language and community come from is met with little more than derision.

   I do not mean to make light of Rorty's impact on contemporary philosophy. His work has unmasked many of the pretensions of academia, as well as the bankruptcy of Anglo-American thought. Yet Rorty does not call into question the presumptions of these very systems, upon which he was nurtured. He appears to be incapable of entertaining foundational options other than those he has so successfully unveiled as fraudulent. There is an unsettled focus in contemporary philosophy that extends far beyond the "decentering" and "marginalizing" work of Foucault and Derrida— although some philosophers regard their projects not so much as an attack on the centrality of the human person as an attack on the atomic and autonomous "man" that was left in the wake of Descartes, the empiricists, and Kant.

   The unsettled condition of contemporary discourse emerges as a prominent theme in a survey of some of the writings of a few prominent recent philosophers in the Anglo-American setting.

Alasdair MacIntyre, in the now-famous *After Virtue* (Notre Dame, Ind.: University of Notre Dame Press, 1984), concludes that "morality today is in a state of grave disorder" (238). This disorder is a result, MacIntyre argues, of the loss of a community of discourse and stability of tradition. He calls for a reinstitution of the Aristotelian tradition (without the metaphysical support that some philosophers would insist is necessary) for the grounding of rational discourse in our moral and social worlds. In *Whose Justice, Which Rationality?* (Notre Dame, Ind.: University of Notre Dame Press, 1989), MacIntyre continues his cautionary searching out of traditions for a suitable foundation for ethics; yet he also continues to avoid confrontation with the reality of the living human person as the foundation of morality and the traditions that demand arbitration between their claims. He makes a great advance, I believe, in correcting this drawback with *Dependent Rational Animals: Why Human Beings Need the Virtues* (Chicago: Open Court, 1999), which not only stresses our continuity with other animals but also explores the possibility of grounding some human virtues in our bodied, animal existence.

After Philosophy: End or Transformation, edited by Kenneth Baynes, James Bohman, and Thomas McCarthy (Cambridge, Mass.: MIT Press, 1988), is a brilliant collection of philosophical pieces that contains the introduction from Rorty's *Consequences of Pragmatism* as well as suggestive pieces by Derrida, Foucault, and Lyotard on the "end of philosophy" and the "end" of the human. These apocalyptic themes are balanced by a range of selections from significant thinkers in communication theory and hermenuetics.

Bernard Williams, in *Ethics and the Limits of Philosophy* (Cambridge, Mass.: Harvard University Press, 1985) is aware of philosophy's loss of confidence; yet Williams offers an invitation to a modest ethical foundation in devotion to the truth and the meaningfulness of an individual's life. Starting with the Socratic question of what one is to do with one's life, he sedulously avoids an investigation into the human person and how the person proposing the question of ethics is constituted to make such a proposal. His values (actually hopes and beliefs) of truth, truthfulness, and the meaning of an individual life—without the foundations in human personhood—can yield only the mix of resignation and hope that marks his fine work. Williams' more recent *Making Sense of Humanity* (New York: Cambridge University Press, 1995) includes several serviceable papers that integrate human identity with moral action.

Richard J. Bernstein, in *Beyond Objectivism and Relativism: Science, Hermeneutics, and Praxis* (Philadelphia: University of Pennsylvania Press, 1983) and *Philosophical Profiles* (New York: Cambridge University Press, 1986), attempts to show that the divisions and poverties of modern philosophical thought are not insurmountable. Bernstein writes with considerable insight and care, aspiring for a reconciled integration—indicated by his dedication to "Four Friends: Hannah Arendt, Hans George Gadamer, Jurgen Habermas, and Richard Rorty." The expanse and inclusiveness of *Beyond Objectivism* may be too optimistic in its unifying promise of a "non-foundational pragmatic humanism" (9), for Bernstein himself is aware of the threat of a "grotesque wild pluralism in which we no longer even know how to communicate with each other" (19) and an uneasy sense of fragmentation at the "giddy whirl of deconstruction in post modern thought" (9, 10).

In *A Theory of Justice* (Cambridge, Mass.: Harvard University Press, 1971), John Rawls offers a more foundational approach to ethics. Rawls has attracted a considerable literature in response to his work, and his book may indeed be the most significant breakthrough in Anglo-American philosophy in the second half of the 20th century—making it respectable, once again, to speak of substantial issues in ethics (as the work of some of his own students has exhibited). The appearance of *A Theory of Justice* in the early 1970s, when I was in graduate school, brought a flood of discussion about topics that had long been repressed by linguistic and logistic scholasticism. Rawls, however, does not investigate the preconditions for his original position—which actually are grounded in convictions about the nature and powers of the human person.

3. I do not intend my complaint about the crisis of contemporary philosophy to slight the substantial contributions of writers such as Bernstein, Rawls, and Macintyre—as well as Martha Nussbaum, Alan Donagan, Margaret Farley, Thomas Nagel, American phenomenologists such as Calvin O. Schrag, personalists, Thomists, and others whom I cite/discuss in subsequent chapters of this book.

   In terms of contemporary philosophical writers, I have found the most challenging and confirming to be Charles Taylor, whose *Sources of the Self: The Making of Modern Identity* (Cambridge, Mass.: Harvard University Press, 1989) has breathtaking range and magisterial depth. Although slight, Taylor's *The Ethics of Authenticity* (Cambridge, Mass.: Harvard University Press, 1991) is an appeal and challenge to diverse philosophical "schools" to admit their own limitations and seek common grounds for discourse.

4. Rorty, *After Philosophy*, 60. Although I have profound reservations about Rorty's philosophy, as well as his influence on contemporary ethical discourse, the writings of Bernstein and Taylor—which I cannot recommend and praise enough—show a capacious appreciation for Rorty's work. Moreover, Rorty has been quite public in his high estimation of Bernstein and Taylor—even when they have been critical of him.

5. Annie Dillard, *For the Time Being* (New York: Alfred Knopf, 1999), 160.

6. Peter Singer, *Rethinking Life and Death: The Collapse of Our Traditional Ethics* (New York: St. Martin's Griffin, 1994), 4. The last sentence of the epigraph quotation appears on page 190.

7. In many ways, the doctrine of the sacredness of human life, though not limited to the Christian tradition, is radicalized in the teachings of Jesus— especially in Matthew 25, in the discourse concerning our treatment of "the least." On the other hand, the absolute inviolability of all human life that I propose in Chapters 6 and 7 of this work may be too extensive an application of nonkilling (i.e., as applied to "the enemy" and "the guilty") for some Christians.

NOTES TO CHAPTER 2

1. Walker Percy, *Lost in the Cosmos* (New York: Washington Square Press, 1983), 256. Percy's book is not just a remarkable satire; it also is the proposal of a philosophical approach to the human person in terms of communication theory and semiotics. Its three segments are an initial set of scenarios that reveal the various pretenses of contemporary American consciousness, a central piece on Percy's theory of signs, and finally a grand fantasy constructed to illuminate our predicament. Although my view of consciousness and human fallenness differs from Percy's, I find it a rare and imaginative treatment of the modern predicament.
2. *Time*, January 16, 1989.
3. Derek Parfit, *Reasons and Persons* (Oxford: Clarendon Press, 1984), 217. Parfit mounts an interesting attack on consequentialist and self-interest theories, convinced that a nonperson-centered ethic will bring less injury to the world. The unasked question that haunts his long treatment is, What is it about persons that they write about themselves and seek out an ethical system? Parfit does not investigate any approach that might be associated with phenomenology, Marxism, or derivatives of the Aristotelian-Thomistic tradition. As a result, his only alternatives are variations of Descartes or Hume.
4. Any characterization of contemporary philosophy, like a characterization of the "African mind" or "Asian consciousness," is hopelessly partial. Although Parfit represents a strong tendency in contemporary philosophy that neglects the lived experience of persons while concentrating on analogies with machines, there is a broad contingent of philosophers—many of whom I mention throughout this book—who confront the perennial personal issues of self-consciousness, body, freedom, anxiety, love, and mortality.

   Even in the field of artificial intelligence, some members of the scientific-cybernetic community wholly reject the identification of machine operations with the human mind. Joseph Weizenbaum, for example, does so in *Computer Power and Human Reason: From Judgment to Calculation* (San Francisco: Freeman, 1976). Weizenbaum mounts an impassioned critique of any "scientism" that somehow postures as being "independent" of the humans who construct it. Science, which is radically dependent on the personal, direct experience of persons, can only be more fallible than the humans who create it. "There is no such thing as mind; there are only individual minds, each belonging, not to 'man,' but to individual human beings. I have argued that intelligence cannot be measured by ingeniously constructed meter sticks placed along a one-dimensional continuum. Intelligence can usefully be discussed only in terms of domains of thought and action. From this I derive the conclusion that it cannot be useful, to say the least, to base serious work on notions of 'how much' intelligence may be given to a computer. Debates based on such ideas—e.g., 'Will computers ever exceed man in intelligence?'—are doomed to sterility" (223).

In more recent years, Marvin Minsky in *Society of Mind* (New York: Simon and Schuster, 1985) had difficulty believing that he has one conscious center, even though he suspected that there may indeed have many little fellows working together in his brain. Daniel Dennett, in the overstatedly titled *Consciousness Explained* (New York: Little and Brown, 1992), would disagree entirely with Weizenbaum's scientific and philosophical rejection of the position that the human mind is a computer. Dennett rightfully notes that his misfortune was to take Descartes so seriously as a college freshman. He roundly rejects Descartes, once again—but only to pose little more than a model of the human mind intimately related to artificial intelligence. A delightful and more popular account of the confused state of reductive "consciousness studies" appears in John Horgan's *The Undiscovered Mind* (New York: Free Press, 1999).

On the other side, Thomas Nagel announced in the March 4, 1993, issue of the *New York Review of Books* that "The Mind Wins." Nagel made the call in his review of John Searle's *The Rediscovery of the Mind* (Cambridge, Mass.: MIT Press, 1993)—a steadfast materialist's *rejection* of reductionism and the computer model of mind. Both philosophers reject any attempt to understand human cognition without a thoroughgoing treatment of consciousness and intentionality. The denial of consciousness does not prove its non existence—especially because every denial rests upon its functioning.

Bioneurologist Gerald Edelman offers an even stronger, more imaginative rejection of any materialist reductionism that neglects the experience of consciousness. *Bright Air, Brilliant Fire: On the Matter of the Mind* (New York: Basic Books, 1992) offers a model of consciousness that is based on an emergent evolutionary model of the human biosystem. Although Edelman's reading of consciousness is not like the one presented in this book, it is wonderfully suggestive and complementary from the viewpoint of "embodiment." Edelman shows how understanding even human memory from the viewpoint of mechanical or computational models alone is impossible.

In terms of academic philosophy, especially with an historical emphasis, one of the preeminent contemporary contributions is Charles Taylor's *Sources of the Self: The Making of Modern Identity* (Cambridge, Mass.: Harvard University Press, 1989), which dramatically expands the perimeters of investigation into human consciousness. Taylor painstakingly prepared for *Sources of the Self* with a series of articles that eventually were collected in a two-volume work. Of particular interest in the current context is the volume of Taylor's philosophical papers titled *Human Agency and Language* (New York: Cambridge University Press, 1985)—a major integration of the human self, courageously resistant to the stereotypes of materialist and spiritualist reductionism.

5. Miguel de Unamuno, *The Tragic Sense of Life* (Princeton, N.J.: Princeton University Press, 1972), 4. One has no doubts where Unamuno stands, where he begins and finishes. He ends his final panegyric to Don Quixote: "And what has Don Quixote left us?. . . . I shall answer that he left us himself. And a man, a living, eternal man, is worth all theories and philosophies. Other nations have bequeathed us, in the main, institutions and books, we have left souls. Teresa of Avila is worth any school or institute, any *Critique of Pure Reason* whatsoever" (350).

6. Rorty, "Pragmatism and Philosophy," in *After Philosophy*, 57.

7. Patricia Churchland, in *Neurophilosophy: Toward a Unified Science of the Mind-Brain* (Cambridge, Mass.: MIT Press, 1986), dismisses the convictions we have about "self-consciousness" as a phenomenon of "folk psychology," ultimately to be replaced by language that has no need for first-person references. The question of whether the "eliminative reductionism" of Churchland and others should bring an end to "folk" theories of self, freedom, love, and so forth has developed into a lively debate. One of the more capacious works is *Folk Psychology and the Philosophy of Mind*, edited by Scott Christensen and Dale Turner (Hillsdale, N.J.: Erlbaum, 1993). A recent powerful challenge by a neurologist to reductionism is Antonio Damasio's *The Feeling of What Happens: Body and Emotion in the Making of Consciousness* (New York: Harcourt, 1999).

8. See the early works of Rollo May—*Love and Will* (New York: Delta, 1964) and *Psychology and the Human Dilemma* (New York: Van Nostrand, 1967)—and the slight but incisive *Freud and Man's Soul*, (New York: Vintage, 1984), as well as Oliver Sacks' *The Man Who Mistook His Wife for a Hat* (New York: Harper & Row, 1984). Similar nonphilosophical treatments of central philosophical issues have been offered by widely differing commentators such as E. F. Schumacher (*Guide for the Perplexed* [New York: Harper & Row, 1977]); Gerald G. May, M.D. (*Will and Spirit: A Contemplative Psychology* [San Francisco: Harper & Row, 1982]); and the uncommonly successful M. Scott Peck, M.D. (*The Road Less Travelled* [New York: Simon and Schuster, 1978]).

Two works of the magisterial Walter Ong are worth particular attention. *Fighting for Life* (Ithaca, N.Y.: Cornell University Press, 1981) is a powerful examination of the constitution of self-identity that has also drawn considerable personal interest by letter and inquiry to the author from feminists, logicians, and semioticians. *Hopkins, the Self and God* (Toronto: Toronto University Press, 1986) is in many ways the key to Ong's spirituality, which undergirds his 50 years of academic labor.

Medicine as well (perhaps because of its ineluctable contact with breathing humans) has taken up the question of human identity—at least in the work of Tristam Engelhardt, Wilder Penfield, Robert Coles, and Sir John Eccles. Most arresting, perhaps, is the work of Oliver Sacks, whose *The Man Who Mistook His Wife for a Hat* is a singularly brilliant apologia for the dignity of the human person.

9. Albert Camus, *The Fall*, trans. Justin O'Brien (New York: Vintage , 1956), 139.

10. Mark Crispin Miller, *Boxed In: The Culture of TV* (Evanston, Ill.: Northwestern University Press, 1988), 330. Miller's brilliant analysis of the latent philosophical themes of the consumer-media culture complements Stuart Ewen's *All Consuming Images* (New York: Basic Books, 1988)—an investigation of a culture defined by style and "surface" and devoted to the domestication of its people. From the perspective of advertising, Eric Clark's *The Want Makers* (New York: Viking, 1989) is a treasure of background and data concerning the surreptitious formation of desires that a given socioeconomic system can muster.

11. Christopher Lasch, *The Minimal Self* (New York: Norton, 1984) and *The Culture of Narcissism* (New York: Norton, 1979). Lasch's *True and Only Heaven* (New York: Norton, 1991) is a brilliant study of historical and cultural disillusionment. It tended to infuriate doctrinaire liberals and conservatives alike—liberals because of his critique of permissiveness, conservatives because of his critique of capitalism. Two more recent—and contrary—accounts of the cultural diminishment of personal life are Robert Frank's *Luxury Fever* (New York: Free Press, 1999) and James Twitchell's *Lead Us Into Temptation* (New York: Columbia University Press, 1999). Frank portrays the cultural and personal impoverishment arising from the consumer culture of excess. Twitchell—in an often hilarious but deadly analysis—celebrates the very loss that Frank mourns.

12. Representative Gary Ackerman, Democrat from New York, reported to the House Education Committee in 1985 that "half a million children try to kill themselves each year, and, tragically, 5,000 of them succeed." *Saint Louis Post-Dispatch*, September 11, 1985.

"For almost all compulsive spenders, the habit causes constant anxiety, guilt and remorse. I often leave the bills sealed for days. . . . I want to beat myself up. I scream, 'No more, I'll never overspend again,' only to repeat the shopping excursions a few days later. The foremost causes are low self-esteem and feelings of powerlessness. . . . 'It's the American Way,' says psychiatrist Dr. Linda Perez, 'but while alcohol shows on your face and body and in your social behavior, debts don't show on the outside.'" "Compulsive Shopping," *Glamour* magazine, April 1986.

The September 15, 1986, cover of *Time* magazine read, "Drugs: The Enemy Within." The sheer dollar volume of narcotics traffic is estimated at anywhere from $27 billion to $110 billion a year. A month earlier, *Newsweek* noted that we have 5 million regular cocaine users.

Estimates of weekly television use range from 27 to 32 hours per week. Most recent data appear in Clark, *The Want Makers*, and Robert McChesney's brilliant *Rich Media Poor Democracy: Communication Politics in Dubious Times* (Urbana: University of Illinois Press, 1999).

13. *Forbes*, September 14, 1992. In September 1986, *Harpers* ran a selection of an article by Christopher Lasch in *Tikkun* in which he discussed the relationship between contemporary culture and the loss of personal mutuality. "It is advertising and the logic of consumerism, not anti-capitalist ideology, that govern the depiction of reality in the media—and, incidentally, tend to undermine 'traditional values.' . . . Even the reporting of news has to be understood . . . as propaganda for commodities—for the replacement of persons by commodities, of events by images. . . . In a society organized around mass consumption, the model of ownership is addiction."

In *Habits of the Heart* (New York: Harper and Row, 1985), Robert Bellah and companions explored the loss of the personal in our communal and civic lives. A reading of this book suggests the paradox—though never making it explicit—that the isolated self-as-individual not only undercuts the possibilities of full personal mutuality but also prevents a fully realized experience of human personhood. This paradox parallels the philosophical paradox that the "isolated monadic self" is neither fully open to inter-subjectivity nor an authentic historically embodied personal self. A valuable companion volume is Bellah et al., *The Good Society* (New York: Knopf, 1991).

14. Syndicated column by Jeffrey Hart, June 27, 1985.

15. Data from Catholic Relief Services, "Facts About World Hunger and World Poverty," and *World Military and Social Expenditures*, 1985 (Box 25140, Washington, D.C., 20007). The childhood mortality statistics are from *Pediatrics* 77, no. 5 (May 1986). In 1984, Dr. Henry Smith noted in *Harvard Magazine* that more American children under five years old are murdered by their parents than die from disease, and more than one million American children are involved in the child pornography industry (with its profit of more than one billion dollars annually).

Columnist George Will in *Newsweek* (February 3, 1997) discussed the tortuous linguistic evasions concerning "partial birth abortion" and infanticide in a bill (HR 1833) that President Bill Clinton vetoed.

16. Personal communication with James Guadalupe Carney, author of *To Be a Revolutionary* (New York: Harper and Row, 1987).

17. Herbert Marcuse, *Five Lectures*, trans. J. Shapiro and S. Weber (Boston: Beacon Press, 1968), 105. In this sentiment, to be sure, Marcuse parted company from other mentors and students of the Frankfurt School (except Erich Fromm—who, as a psychoanalytic Marxist, adopted a modified natural law theory in some of his ethical works). Adorno and Horkheimer surely would have found this "essentialist" turn in their offspring scandalous.

18. Calvin Schrag, in his introduction to *Communicative Praxis and the Space of Subjectivity* (Bloomington: Indiana University Press, 1989), makes this very point while noting that traces of subjectivity remain even after the most direct attacks on it.

19. Alasdair MacIntyre, *Whose Justice? Which Rationality?* (Notre Dame, Ind.: University of Notre Dame Press, 1988), 367.

20. Alasdair MacIntyre, *Dependent Rational Animals* (Chicago: Open Court, 1999).

21. Pierre Manent has argued in *The City of Man* (Princeton, N.J.: Princeton University Press, 1998) that the isolated emphasis on consciousness in history has unmoored humanity from its anchor in nature. Autonomy and Self are exclusively affirmed at the cost of our connectedness—not only with nature but with each other.

As for Rorty, he is bold in his refusal to consider the "self," the "person," or the "I." In *Contingency, Irony and Solidarity* (New York: Cambridge University Press, 1989), he champions the assertion that there is no such thing as "human nature" or "the deepest level of the self." For Rorty, the nature of the human person is an unprofitable topic. Discussing the "contingencies of selfhood," he praises Freud for having abandoned "the very idea of a paradigm human being. He does not see humanity as a natural kind with an intrinsic nature, an intrinsic set of powers to be developed or left undeveloped" (35). This reading of Freud is debatable. Surely, Freud's hermeneutics of suspicion mounts an impressive attack on the pretenses of the false self or overly facile notions of human natural endowments—especially autonomous reason. But Freud, willy nilly, *has* a doctrine of human nature as well as human endowments as conditions even for the possibility of therapy and psychiatric hermeneutics.

Despite Rorty's high visibility, ingenuity, and impact on the most recent of philosophical discussions, his positions have not gone unquestioned. In "Rortyism," *Philosophy and Literature* 12, no. 1 (April 1988): 27–47, Martin Steinman not only playfully notes that Rorty himself has a doctrine of human nature; he also shows how Rorty's notion of language suffers from a lack of any grounding or any criteria for arbitrating language claims. Doris Leland, "Rorty on the Moral Concern of Philosophy: A Critique from a Feminist Point of View" and Nancy Fraser, "Solidarity or Singularity? Richard Rorty Between Romanticism and Technocracy"—both in *Praxis International* 8 (October 1988)—offer reservations from a feminist perspective. Perhaps the most telling critique has been offered by Thomas McCarthy in "Private Irony and Public Decency: Richard Rorty's New Pragmatism," *Critical Inquiry* 16 (Winter 1990): 355–70. McCarthy offers a powerful challenge to Rorty from a Habermasian and leftist background. This challenge was telling enough that it appeared as the subject of the last chapter of *Prospects for a Common Morality*, edited by Gene Outka and John Reeder (Princeton, N.J.: Princeton University Press, 1993), 279–89. This chapter features Rorty's not entirely compelling self-defense, "Truth and Freedom: A Reply to Thomas McCarthy."

22. An excellent survey of American phenomenology appears in the *Analecta Husserliana*, Vol. 26, edited by E. F. Kaelin and C. O. Schrag (Boston: Kluwer Academic Publishers, 1989). This survey provides a strong sense of the vibrant diversity in just this one corridor in the house of American philosophy. Among the valuable historical accounts and personal entries is that of James Marsh, whose *Post-Cartesian Meditations* (New York: Fordham, 1988) is an attempt to ground "authentic selfhood" through a politically critical and phenomenological hermeneutic of the human person which is neither Cartesian not mechanistic. In neo-Thomist and personalist circles, Jacques Maritain and Emmanuel Mounier continue to exercise strong influence. James Hanink, "The Personalist Vision," *New Oxford Review*, March 1989, 6–11, offers a recent reflection.

23. Habermas—his own career an impressive range of labors integrating Hegelian Marxism, communication theory, language, and neo-Kantianism— may be the preeminent international figure who promises to overcome of the chasm between Anglo-American and European philosophy. Although he carefully avoids "searching out of the foundations" in any substantive view of the human person, a case can be made that his theory of communicative action and the conditions underlying it not only provide a philosophical approach that transcends cultural confinement but also require a doctrine of human nature.

24. Richard Bernstein, *The New Constellation: The Ethical-Political Horizons of Modernity/Postmodernity* (Cambridge, Mass.: MIT Press, 1991), 164. The earlier point is made on page 146, in reference to Foucault's discussion on the Enlightenment.

   In addition to Bernstein, whose *Beyond Objectivism and Relativism* and *Philosophical Profiles* have contributed much to the opening and expanding of philosophical discussions, Thomas Nagel—especially in *Mortal Questions* (New York: Cambridge University Press, 1979) and *The View From Nowhere* (New York: Oxford University Press, 1986)—has boldly and imaginatively cracked open the confining perimeters of philosophy-talk in the United States. Lawrence E. Cahoone, *The Dilemma of Modernity* (Albany, N.Y.: SUNY Press, 1988) also seeks to reopen questions of the person in the broader contexts of intersubjectivity and culture.

25. Calvin O. Schrag, *Experience and Being* (Evanston, Ill.: Northwestern University Press, 1969), 15–22. Wittgenstein offered a less abstract way of insisting on the concrete experiential starting point in a letter to Russell: "Perhaps you regard this thinking about myself as a waste of time—but how can I be a logician before I'm a human being!" *Letters to Russell, Keynes and Moore* (Ithaca, N.Y.: Cornell University Press, 1974), 58.

NOTES TO CHAPTER THREE

1. Derek Parfit, *Reasons and Persons* (Oxford: Clarendon Press, 1984), 275, 279.

2. Sacks, *The Man Who Mistook His Wife for a Hat*, 124. Among Sacks' many publications is an account of traumatic memory loss and recovery in *Awakenings* (New York: Harper Perennial, 1990)—an uncommonly moving clinical study that reveals the dialectic of self-consciousness and body. Sacks is influenced by the life and work of Anton Luria and Luria's call for a new "personalistic" and "romantic" science of neurology.

3. Maurice Merleau-Ponty, *The Essential Writings of Merleau-Ponty*, ed. Alden L. Fisher (New York: Harcourt, Brace and World, 1969), 141–42. The selection is from *The Structure of Behavior* (Boston: Beacon Press, 1963), Chapter 4, 185–224.

4. Parfit, *Reasons and Persons*, 216. The same constraint is in Peter Carruthers' *Introducing Persons* (Albany, N.Y.: SUNY Press, 1986): "The Dualist holds that the person, or self, should be identified with the soul" (40). This is the *only* position, consequently, that Carruthers exposes as inadequate.

   Kathleen Wilkes, in *Real People: Personal Identity without Thought Experiments* (Oxford: Clarendon Press, 1988), chides philosophers who seem under the spell of science-fiction concoctions. Her initial quarrel with the excessive use of thought experiments is not only because they neglect our "lived," ordinary world and our common sense. She is more seriously concerned with the substantial claim—grounded in Aristotle's notion of the soul—that the human is a dynamic unity whose activities are informed by the soul. Psyche is not some "mind" or hermetic "self"; it is the soul of the whole acting being. Wilkes mounts a strong criticism of Descartes, Locke, and Hume for collapsing the notion of the self, the psyche, or the soul into the *mens* or "consciousness." Her warnings are well worth heeding for any reader of this book—especially those who think its emphasis on reflexive consciousness is dualistic or somehow identifies the "self" with "awareness of awareness."

James Baillie, whose *Problems in Personal Identity* (New York: Paragon House, 1993) is a short evaluation of Parfit's work, also has read Kathleen Wilkes. Baillie seems not to have taken her warnings seriously, however. He has a fascination with the brain-as-self, apparently agreeing with Thomas Nagel that "I go where my brain goes." Again, the dynamic unity of a human person is ignored. In a brain transplant, for instance, the most accurate judgment is that *both* original persons have died. What survives is a seriously damaged, newly constructed person. No doubt we can tamper with an individual's sense of identity by brain surgery—or drugs, beer, or lead paint, for that matter. This fact is not in question. What is in question is the status of the new hybrid. Most observers would judge that there would be greater continuity with the previous owner of the brain—at least in terms of possible mental states. I do not think it is that easy. Imagine the brain of a 30-year-old male dwarf transplanted into the body of a 12-year-old girl.

5. The alternative? "What a reductionist denies is that the subject of experience is a *separately* existing entity *distinct* from a brain and body, and a series of physical and mental events" (Parfit, *Reason and Persons*, 223) and "Suppose that the cause of psychological continuity was not the continued existence of the brain, but the continued existence of a *separately existing* entity, like a Cartesian ego" (*Ibid.*, 237). (I have emphasized what I am precisely *not* claiming in this book.)

In *The Mind and Its World* (London: Routledge, 1995), Gregory McCulloch—writing under the influence of Wittgenstein and phenomenology—sees the residual Cartesianism of the new "brain science" and its neglect of the lived experience of what it is like to be a human. Rejecting the false option between a "disembodied mind" (Descartes) and a "disembodied brain" (the new materialism), McCulloch proposes a view of embodiment that avoids the dogmas of scientism. The lived experience of humans cannot be repressed merely because it is unexplained by material reductionism. McCullough's final sentence is: "To destroy something because you don't understand it is simply to lapse into barbarism" (220).

6. Similar doubts about inadequate maps, it seems, have led Nagel and others to more directly face the conflicts in the false dichotomy of mind and brain. In the painfully honest *The View From Nowhere* (a title preeminently and provocatively appropriate) (New York: Oxford University Press, 1986), Nagel refuses to repress any evidence that might challenge either the reductionist or the nonreductionist position. Because he sees the alter-

natives, however, as a strange, disembodied, unhistorical sense of subjectivity versus an equally strange, impersonal, dead sense of objectivity, the book is largely a confession of failure in reconciling the various antinomies of human existence. In effect, Nagel offers something of a truce between two domains of truth. I propose, however, that it is one truth from the beginning: the truth of an embodiment as paradoxical as human existence itself is. Nagel reaches for this truth in affirmations such as "we are first of all and essentially individual human beings" (221). He also is convinced that the reductionist program "that dominates current work in the philosophy of mind is completely misguided" because of its objectivist presumptions and its fascination with computer analogies (16). The absence of a full theory of embodiment or dynamic nature prevents him, however, from arriving at a possible answer to our greatest need: "What is needed is something we do not have: a *theory of conscious organisms* as physical systems composed of chemical elements and occupying space, which also have an individual perspective on the world, and in some cases a *capacity for self-awareness as well*. In some way that we do not now understand, our minds as well as our bodies come into being when these materials are suitably combined and organized. The strange truth seems to be that certain complex, biologically generated physical systems, of which each of us is an example, have rich *nonphysical* properties. An integrated theory of reality must account for this, and I believe that if and when it arrives, probably not for centuries, it will alter our conception of the universe as anything has to date" (51). The emphasis is mine.

7. This is a mark of much philosophy that comes out of the Anglo-American analytic tradition. Although I do not think that "thought experiments" are essentially misleading or a waste of time, I do find puzzling that such weight—even at the earliest stages of investigation—is given to these fantasies when there is so little discussion or tolerance of phenomenological procedures. See Daniel C. Dennett, *Brainstorms: Philosophical Essays on Mind and Psychology* (Cambridge, Mass.: MIT Press, 1986). See also Rorty's discussion of the "Antipodeans" in the "Persons Without Minds" chapter of *Philosophy and the Mirror of Nature*. Note as well the absence of any phenomenological recognition and the abundance of thought experiments in Bernard Williams' *Problems of the Self* (New York: Cambridge University Press, 1976). The fine scholarship of this book, as narrow as some might have found it to be, is remarkably opened up in Williams' equally incisive but far more experiential *Ethics and the Limits of Philosophy* (Cambridge, Mass.: Harvard University Press, 1985). Written with more compelling immediacy, it locates the ethical enterprise in the Socratic questions of human identity and praxis and remains profoundly personalized until the end. Finally, although Amelie Rorty's *Mind in Action* (Boston: Beacon Press, 1988) has a profound sense of litera-

ture, drama, and history, it exhibits a fateful tendency toward human
model-options as disembodied selves or entirely socialized products. She
also stands in the tradition of utter fascination for thought experiments
about damaged humans. Yet one would think that one need not look to the
science fiction scenarios of the second half of the 20th century to see that
personal identity is a fragile thing. Even a change in diet, much more sense
deprivation, has a profound impact on personal identity. One does not need
a brain transplant fantasy to get the point across.

8. The extended discussion is in David Hume, *A Treatise of Human Nature*, Book
I, Part IV, Section VI (1739). Hume cannot find an impression that yields
the self, only that "when I enter most intimately into what I call *myself*, I always stumble on some particular perception or other. . . . I never can catch
myself at any time without a perception." As we shall see, the "entering"
done by the "I" as the condition of possibility for the expedition is at issue.
William Barrett, in *The Death of the Soul* (New York: Doubleday, 1986), 46,
suggested that Hume's maneuver is similar to the man who went outside
his house and looked in the window to see if he was in there.

9. Sacks, *The Man Who Mistook His Wife for a Hat*, 125.

10. Merleau-Ponty, *The Essential Writings*, 369 ("A Prospectus of His Work").

11. Antonio Damasio, *The Feeling of What Happens: Body and Emotion in the Making
of Consciousness* (New York: Harcourt, Brace & Co., 1999), 40.

12. *Ibid.*, 347, footnote 4. Damasio also points out, in his own way, the paradoxical nature of embodiment that I address. "When creatures like us appeared, which had bodies and conscious minds, they were, as Nietzsche
would call them, 'hybrids of plants and of ghosts,' the combination of a
bounded, well circumscribed, easily identifiable living object with a seemingly unbounded, internal, and difficult-to-localize mental animation. He
also called these creatures 'discords,' for they did possess a strange marriage of the clearly material with the apparently insubstantial. The marriage has puzzled everyone for millennia, and now may be, to some extent,
a little easier to understand than before. Maybe" (142). A lovely humility.

13. Calvin Schrag clearly has this inescapable subjectivity, always contextual,
in mind throughout *Communicative Praxis and the Space of Subjectivity* (Bloomington: Indiana University Press, 1986), the effort of which is this: "The
subject as speaker, author, and actor is restored, not as a foundation for
communicative praxis but as an implicate of it. Implicated within the dynamics of communicative praxis the subject emerges via its co-constitution
with other subjects as the narrator, actor, and respondent within the
human drama of discourse and social praxis" (138). In Schrag's Introduction, he reminds us that even so "decentering" a "deconstructionist" as
Derrida admitted in a discussion that "the subject is absolutely indispensable: I don't destroy the subject. I situate it. That is to say, I believe that at a

certain level both of experience and of philosophical and scientific discourse one cannot get along without the notion of subject. It is a question
of knowing where it comes from and how it functions" (10–11). Schrag's
work, to which I am indebted, is summarized in *The Self after Postmodernity*
(New Haven, Conn.: Yale University Press, 1997), where he defends the
human as "incarnate consciousness of the self as embodied" (53).

14. Damasio, *The Feeling of What Happens*, 10.

15. Gilbert Ryle, *The Concept of Mind* (New York: Barnes and Noble, 1949), 11.
    At the end of this work, Ryle says its purpose was to show that the
    two-worlds story is a philosophers' myth and to repair the damage that this
    myth caused philosophy. One might fully agree with the goal, yet believe
    that the greatest damage has been done by those who suppose that the
    only option to behaviorism and mind-brain identity theory is that of the
    Cartesian myth. The hard dichotomy between consciousness and world
    leads to a view from nowhere.

    The work of Charles Taylor can be regarded as an attempt to offer
    something other than the "forced options" of pure subjectivity and pure
    objectivity. In *Human Agency and Language* (New York: Cambridge Univer-
    sity Press, 1985), Taylor notes that his efforts have a polemical concern: "I
    wanted to argue against the understanding of human life and action im-
    plicit in an influential family of theories in the sciences of man. The com-
    mon feature of this family is the ambition to model the study of man on the
    natural sciences. Theories of this kind seem to me to be terribly implausi-
    ble. They lead to very bad science: Either they end up in wordy elabora-
    tions of the obvious, or they fail altogether to address the interesting ques-
    tions, or their practitioners end up squandering their talents and ingenuity
    in the attempt to show that they can after all recapture the insights of ordi-
    nary life in their manifestly reductive explanatory languages" (1).

16. Aquinas—whom many people might unwittingly accuse of a medieval "du-
    alism" that has the soul residing as some autonomous and separate inner
    substance-self—was insistent that the soul was not the self, nor the person,
    nor the "true man." In fact, for Aquinas, the soul upon death could only be
    understood as an "incomplete" substance—not even a true individual real-
    ity on its own, so essential to its identity was its embodied condition as a
    historical human unity. In the *Summa Theologica*, for example, he says,
    "Since the soul is united to the body as form and as a natural component of
    human nature, its creation does not precede its union with the body. By
    creation God constitutes things in the perfection of their nature. Apart
    from the body, the soul lacks its natural perfection, and it would be awk-
    ward for it to be created in this condition" (Ia, xc, 4).

17. Soren Kierkegaard, *The Sickness Unto Death*, trans. Walter Lowrie (Prince-
    ton, N.J.: Princeton University Press, 1951), 17.

18. The phenomenon of reflexive consciousness equated with "the self" is a pervasive tendency not only in Kierkegaard but in many others who have made efforts to discuss the phenomenon. Pure reflexivity, without content, is not done by any embodied human being. For this reason, we are in some ways always unknown to ourselves, always in some ways opaque and undiscovered. The process of growing self-understanding, self-possession, and self-disposition is made possible, however, by the pure reflexivity of consciousness—an act of the person, but not the person. To hold otherwise is to fall on the Cartesian side of Ryle's forced alternative.

19. Although it valorizes the social and linguistic components in the formation of individual personal identity, Ron Harre's *Personal Being* (Cambridge, Mass.: Harvard University Press, 1984) attempts to disengage personal identity and morality from the hegemony of positive science and the artificial intelligence model—as well as the Cartesian variations of the pure thinking self. Harre's work is marked by excellent and wide-ranging bibliographies and project proposals for further investigation.

    In the field of social science, Anthony Giddens has been possibly the most comprehensive theoretician. His *Modernity and Self-Identity: Self and Society in the Late Modern Age* (Stanford, Calif.: Stanford University Press, 1991) emphasizes the active and passive components of the individual's relationship to the social world. Giddens has a strong notion of "reflexivity" in the self and a commitment to the ethical implications in a theory of self: "Personal meaninglessness—the feeling that life has nothing worthwhile to offer—becomes a fundamental psychic problem in the circumstances of late modernity. We should understand this phenomenon in terms of a repression of moral questions which day-to-day life poses, but which are denied answers" (9).

20. Gerard Manley Hopkins, *The Poems of Gerard Manley Hopkins*, ed. W. H. Gardner and N. H. MacKenzie (Oxford: Oxford University Press, 1970), 90.

21. "The higher a nature, the more intimate what comes from it, for its inwardness of activity corresponds to its rank in being. . . . The supreme and perfect grade of life is found in mind, which can reflect on itself and understand itself." Thomas Aquinas, *Summa contra Gentiles*, IV, II.

22. It is frustrating, for example, that Churchland's impressive 545-page *Neurophilosophy* makes no attempt to discuss the phenomenon of reflexive consciousness.

23. Jean-Paul Sartre, in *The Transcendence of the Ego*, trans. Forrest Williams and Robert Kirkpatrick (New York: Octagon Books, 1972), grapples with the relationship between pure reflexive consciousness as a transcendental field and the bodied-self. Sartre's strong dualistic identification of the *pour soi* with human reality has unfortunate implications not only for intersub-

jectivity but for human biology and ethics as well. In contrast, Damasio extends the notion of self down to the level of any organized integrated systems (proto-selves), quite amenable to evolutionary biology. He also distinguishes a "core" self from the autobiographical self (*The Feeling of What Happens*, 64–65). I believe that reflexive consciousness represents a quantum leap from lower levels of consciousness.

24. Wilder Penfield, in *The Mystery of the Mind* (Princeton, N.J.: Princeton University Press, 1975), writes how his probing of the cortex in grand mal patients led him to the discovery that memory bits are highly specified and localizable. Penfield's work is a remarkable confirmation of the Aristotelian contention that the cortex was the actual organ of memory as well as the other "internal sense" activities of sense unification, sense evaluation, and sense imagination:

> For example, when a mother told me she was suddenly aware, as my electrode touched the cortex, of being in her kitchen listening to the voice of her little boy who was playing outside in the yard. She was aware of the neighborhood noises, such as passing motor cars, that might mean danger to him. . . . D. F. could hear instruments playing a melody. I re-stimulated the same point thirty times trying to mislead her, and dictated each response to a stenographer. Each time I re-stimulated, she heard the melody again. It began at the same place and went on from chorus to verse" (21–22).

Penfield recommends a dualism that I find as unconvincing as the materialism of his opposition. In light of work by Oliver Sacks and Gerald Edelman and by Damasio, even his notion of memory is is too spatialized and mechanical.

25. *Ibid.*, 55.

26. Richad Restak, M.D., *The Mind* (New York: Bantam, 1988), 29–31.

27. More anecdotally, an Associated Press story in spring 1981 carried a report concerning a Minneapolis policeman whom doctors described as being in a "persistent vegetative state" for most of 1980. After being shot in the brain, officer David Mack was observed as having no interaction at all with his environment. Yet after he "regained" consciousness and became capable of communicating through a word-board, he revealed that for a while he thought he was dead. Later, he thought he was in hell. We have here a person, a self, whose encounter of the world is frighteningly altered by the damage the "whole" person suffers. The "stream" of the content of consciousness is so radically diminished that Officer Mack thinks that he (himself) is dead and then experiences a condition that can only be described as hellish. Throughout much of this experience, however, he has a reflexive consciousness that appropriates these tragic deficits as his own. The question of his identity persists. The question of what attitude and stance he

might take toward the world remains. The human person—embodied awareness of awareness, damaged though the body may be—endures. An article in the *Chicago Tribune* on March 22, 1983, again noted this account, describing the depression that Mack was fighting as a resident of a nursing home for disabled adults. Although this is anecdotal testimony from the popular press, can we not give it the same weight as thought experiments?

With regard to sensory deficits, Helen Keller's *The Story of My Life* (New York: Airmont Books, 1965), 20–23 and 186–87, gives a stirring account of human self-consciousness, capable of and desirous of affirmation, unable to appropriate the instrumentality of spoken or signed language because she lost sight and hearing in infancy.

The most fascinating split-brain operations are recounted in Eileen P. G. Vining et al., "Why Would You Remove Half a Brain? The Outcome of 58 Children After Hemispherectomy—the Johns Hopkins Experience: 1968 to 1996," *Pediatrics* 100, no. 2 (August 1997): 163–71. One of the cases, which involved a girl in her early teens named Cassie, was the topic of a subsequent story on *Dateline NBC*. With half her brain removed, not only was Cassie fully conscious of herself as a self, she eventually recovered the affective integration of her bright personality, speech, and physical movement.

NOTES TO CHAPTER FOUR

1. "Just Like Us," *Harpers* magazine, August 1988, 49.
2. Universal Declaration of Human Rights, Article One.
3. Thomas Aquinas, *Summa contra Gentiles*, IV, II.
4. Indeed, there are epistemological issues that might be raised. The appeal to some received wisdom that knowing what a substance or a nature might be is impossible must be supported, however, by arguments that rest on experience—not merely the epistemological grid offered by Descartes or Hume. I have stopped counting the times when I have been reminded, "Obviously, no one can hold that there are natural kinds anymore" and when I ask for the reasons why, I am given nothing other than stillness or the resonance of long-held dogma. I will be the first to admit, however, that a full-blown philosophy of the human person and ethics requires epistemological and metaphysical support as much as it requires available data from psychology and neuroscience.
5. The whole issue here is whether we can characterize humans as radically different in kind from other animals. If humans act in radically different ways and are thereby radically different in their capacities or endowments, one can justify treating humans in a different way. Ultimately, the debate over animal rights and "speciesism" will come down to such issues. Peter Singer's original 1975 defense of animal rights has been more recently ed-

ited in *Animal Liberation* (New York: New York Review, 1990). He empha-sizes activated sentience, rather than endowed personhood.

Among the places one might look for treatments of animal communica-tion are *How Animals Communicate* (Bloomington: Indiana University Press, 1977), edited by Thomas Sebeok—who also put together the critical an-thology *Speaking of Apes* (New York: Plenum, 1980). Jane Goodall's power-fully empathetic account in *Through a Window: My Thirty Years with the Chim-panzees of Gombe* (Boston: Houghton Mifflin, 1990) contrasts with Herbert Terrace's more critical *Nim: A Chimpanzee Who Learned Sign Language* (New York: Knopf, 1979). More recently, Dorothy Cheney and Robert Seyfarth make a strong case for human-nonhuman continuities in *How Monkeys See the World: Inside the Mind of Another Species* (Chicago: University of Chicago Press, 1990). A quite different approach is Stephen Budiansky's *If A Lion Could Talk* (New York: The Free Press, 1998). (The lion would have noth-ing personal to say.)

Might "rights" also be extended to machines? For approaches that are far different than that of this book, see Hans Moravec, *Mind Children: The Future of Robot and Human Intelligence* (Cambridge, Mass.: Harvard University Press, 1988), and Sherry Turkle, *The Second Self: Computers and the Human Spirit* (New York: Touchstone Books, 1984).

Two more popular accounts of the differences among human, animals, and machines are Alan Wolfe's *The Human Difference* (Berkeley: University of California Press, 1993)—written from a sociologist's perspective—and physicist James Trefil's *Are We Unique: A Scientist Explores the Unparalleled Intelli-gence of the Human Mind* (New York: Wiley and Sons, 1997).

6. Walter Ong has a telling observation on the absence of self-communica-tive depth in animals. Ong says that perhaps animals have never been found to "say" anything because they have nothing to say. "Every human person who is physiologically and psychologically mature can say 'I' and does. Other living beings quite evidently cannot do this. It is naive to say that maybe they can, only we cannot tell, as some have said of the pongid apes. For one of the quite evident paradoxes of the self-conscious self, which 'I' expresses, is that, although it is directly accessible only from its interior to itself—only I know what it feels like to be me—it is irresistibly driven to make itself known exteriorly, to other self-consciousnessess. If a chimpanzee could say 'I,' you can be sure that he or she would let other 'I's hear of his or her 'I' without delay. A self-conscious self is desperately con-cerned to make sure that other selves can tell that it knows itself. Other-wise, other selves treat it as a thing, an exterior, not as the reflexive interior that it is, and this a self, a person, cannot bear, for such treatment equiva-lently denies the self its very existence." *Hopkins, the Self, and God* (Toronto: University of Toronto Press, 1986), 36.

7. The "mirror" notion of reflexive consciousness is evident from the title of Rorty's *Philosophy and the Mirror of Nature*. It also haunts the work of countless others, including Derrida. Rodolphe Gasche's incisive and stimulating study, *The Tain of the Mirror* (Cambridge, Mass.: Harvard University Press, 1986), is itself, like Derrida's deconstructions, mounted on the misunderstanding that the reflexivity of consciousness is something like a mirror that reflects. The experience of awareness of awareness is nothing like seeing oneself in a mirror. It is more accurately understood by the analogy of a mirror that would both be itself and behind itself seeing through itself the content of the world. *Cf.* 20–21 and 82–23.

8. Percy, *Lost in the Cosmos*, 165. The issue of "immateriality" in reflexive consciousness will be further challenged, of course, as research in artificial intelligence and animal behavior progresses. If research shows that computers have reflexive consciousness, the implication will be that such an act is materially-electronically based. It also will suggest, on the account offered here, that because such machines would be capacitated for freedom and love, they would be persons. The same conclusions would apply to nonhuman animals.

9. Colin McGinn, *The Mysterious Flame: Conscious Minds in a Material World* (New York: Basic Books, 1999), 14.

10. *Ibid.*, 47. The citation is from page 60.

11. There is an impressive spectrum of nonreductive work on the "mind-body." John Searle's latest, *Mind, Language and Society: Philosophy in the Real World* (New York: Basic Books, 1998), cogently summarizes his attempts to honor the biological basic of human experience while insisting on the non-reducibility of consciousness. Bernard Baars, *In The Theater of Consciousness* (New York: Oxford University Press, 1997), offers a more scientific but accessible integration of neurology, biology, and experiential selfhood. Eleonore Stump, "Non-Cartesian Substance Dualism and Materialism without Reductionism," *Faith and Philosophy* 12, no. 4 (October 1995): 505–30, offers a more specifically analytic and philosophical contemporary reading of Aquinas.

12. Thus, for Sartre, human freedom somehow precedes human essence or what the human is. Sartre's critique of determinism in *Being and Nothingness* remains remarkably effective, yet his radical separation of the *pour soi* from the *en soi* is so inextricably dualist that the kind of freedom he proposes is precisely a freedom that falls so easily before the determinist assault. See *Being and Nothingness*, trans. Hazel Barnes (New York: Washington Square Press, 1966), 533–38.

13. In *Science and Human Behavior* (New York: Macmillan, 1953), 447, Skinner claims that the notion of the "free inner man" is a "prescientific substitute" for the causes of human behavior, all of which lie outside the individual.

Almost two decades later, in *Beyond Freedom and Dignity* (New York: Bantam-Vintage, 1971)—where he develops more extensively the philosophical background of his position—Skinner clearly indicates that the "inner man" is not at all the self given phenomenologically in experience. Instead, it is the Cartesian self again, an "autonomous man" because "his behavior is uncaused" (see 11–20).

14. Freud makes this clear in his meta-psychological writings, his lectures, and his view of therapy. Thus, in *The Future of an Illusion* (New York: Norton, 1961), he insists that "the voice of intellect is a soft one, but it does not rest till it has gained a hearing. Finally, after a countless succession of rebuffs, it succeeds" (53). Therefore he can claim, at the end of the book, that his "science is not an illusion" (56). "Intellect," as Freud uses the term, has as its foundation and condition for possibility "awareness of awareness," as I have described it.

    Paul Ricoeur, in *Freud and Philosophy: An Essay on Interpretation* (New Haven, Conn.: Yale University Press, 1970), notes that the humbling of the Ego is achieved precisely in the new breakthrough of self-understanding (427). Finally, in the stirring conclusion to the 31st lecture in *New Introductory Lectures on Psycho-Analysis*, Freud unveils the goal of therapy: "For their object is to strengthen the Ego, to make it more independent of the Super-ego, to widen its field of vision, and so to extend its organization that it can take over new portions of the Id. Where Id was, there shall Ego be" (see any edition, end of Lecture 31). Again, the conscious rationality that serves as the force for liberation in the Ego, has for its condition of possibility the act of concomitant reflexive awareness.

15. Merleau-Ponty. *The Essential Writings*, 136. This idea is quite similar to Ricoeur's notion of a "mere human freedom that is motivated, incarnate, contingent" developed in his philosophy of will and reconfirmed in *Freud and Philosophy*, 458.

16. Helen Keller, *The Story of My Life.*

17. Colin McGinn, *Minds and Bodies: Philosophers and Their Ideas* (New York: Oxford University Press, 1997), 220. The options for other kinds of persons are suggested by the citation from Aquinas at the beginning of the chapter, in which he writes of minds that know themselves. Thus, just as questions are raised about whether there may be personal minds in nonhuman animals or computers, so also the question may be raised whether there may be disembodied "spirits" or pure minds or angels—or even an absolute mind.

18. Thus, one might have a view of the self as socially constituted, or as "fully functioning," or as discoverable only in relationship. One also might see the self as emergent only with maturation. I believe that the biological, developmental, social, and genetic evidence corresponds to my own use of

the term "self" to indicate the whole human career. I choose this usage to indicate the conditions for the possibility of a human self's origin, elaboration, and ending throughout an embodied, awareness-of-awareness continuum.

19. Boethius, *De Persona et duabus naturis*, Ch. 3; PL 64: 1345.

20. C. S. Lewis in *Studies in Words* (New York: Cambridge University Press, 1960) offers a helpful discussion of the word "nature" in relation to "*phusis*" and "kind." His characterization helps us understand the relationship between nature and dynamic process—in the original moment of self-development and in its termination of the natural being's capacity to act (24–75). Christopher Berry offers a contemporary treatment in *Human Nature* (Atlantic, N.J.: Humanities Press, 1986). This compact, cogent, yet wide-ranging treatment of the notion from ethical and political perspectives is cognizant of recent debates.

21. The relation between essence and nature may be at the basis of this misunderstanding because the word *essence* is much more susceptible to static interpretation and application. In his little essay *Being and Essence*, Aquinas offers a remarkable discussion of the various meanings of *essence* and notes that in relationship to "nature," *essence* has a marked dynamic quality.

22. Abraham Maslow discusses this phenomenon in the context of basic propositions for a self-actualization philosophy. In *Toward a Psychology of Being*, 2nd ed. (Princeton, N.J.: Van Nostrand Insight Books, 1962), 189–94, Maslow presents a notion of human nature as uniquely capacitated and subject to developmental influence. This nature is discovered, not invented. It is basically good and to be "followed." If one is unfaithful to this nature or if it is suppressed by others, one becomes dysfunctional.

    Although not a natural law theorist, James Q. Wilson in *The Moral Sense* (New York: Free Press, 1993) provides, from a biosociological perspective, a reading of human nature that is constant over times and cultures but fragile and open to environmental conditioning.

23. Having a human nature with endowed capacities, therefore, is indeed a determinant (and to this extent, it is a "cause" of human free action). The paradox, however, is that a distinctive endowment of such a being is that it is open, not rigidly programmed to be and act out what it is. What kind of being is a human? A kind of being that does not *have* to be the kind of being it is.

24. Wilkes, in *Real People*, takes on this issue: "The 'Aristotelian principle' broadly claims that every creature strives after its own perfection, and thus that any member of kind K is in some respect something to be pitied or deplored. The stunted oak is a failure as an oak—it is not all it might be. The puppy born with a twisted paw is deplored by the tough-minded and pitied by the tender-minded, even though it may be just as content, and in other

respects as healthy, as its unimpaired siblings" (62). Wilkes is working here with a notion not only of capacity or endowment but also of natural kind—something between "stringent essentialism and loose conventionalism."

Anthony Kenny's excellent *The Metaphysics of Mind* (Oxford: Clarendon Press, 1989)—written in the spirit of Gilbert Ryle but by a Wittgensteinian Thomist—has a particularly interesting chapter (Chapter 5) that deals with the notions we have been discussing, especially "abilities" and "faculties." Kenny's work is especially valuable for professional philosophers who are unfamiliar with Aquinas and for beginning philosophers who wish to investigate the Thomist tradition.

One hopes that in the future, works by writers such as Wilkes and Kenny will be more closely inspected by philosophers who are investigating the "mind-body" problem. For example, although the fine study by Owen Flanagan, *Consciousness Reconsidered* (Cambridge: MIT Press, 1992), is conversant with some of Wilkes, Flanagan seems to be unaware of Kenny's efforts. This lack of breadth is what leads to forced restricted options between models of the mind as well as a too-frequent caricature of nonreductionistic positions. Flanagan's sources are heavily weighted toward mechanistic, materialistic, and reductionistic models, although he is to be commended for resisting the smug suggestions of some thinkers that "consciousness" is irrelevant unless one is doing something like "folk" psychology. Flanagan's treatment of the brain is cogent and uncommonly clear; his acknowledgment of consciousness is welcome: "I conclude that subjective awareness plays a role in our mental lives. But exactly what role it plays, how important it is in fixing informational content, in what domains it is important, how it figures in remembering, what its relation is to attention, whether it is constitutive of certain kinds of sensation and memory, or whether it receives output from the sensory modules and memory—all these are unsettled questions. Until they are settled, the precise roles of subjective awareness will remain unclear, as will its relative importance in the multifarious domains of mental life" (151). This humility is appropriate.

25. The example is from an actual case. This is the most recent of many accounts of emergence from extended coma and "permanent vegetative state." On Christmas Eve 1999, Patricia White Bull became suddenly alert after 16 years in coma caused by brain damage from oxygen deficiency while she was giving birth. Although she was classified as vegetative, there were no data about where she had registered, for example, on the Glasgow Coma Scale. The Associated Press story appeared, among other places, in the *Saint Louis Post-Dispatch*, January 5, 2000, A4.

26. Evelyn B. Pluhar, *Beyond Prejudice* (Durham, N.C.: Duke University Press, 1995), 83. Pluhar's argument is essentially repeated in McGinn's *Minds and Bodies* and Daniel Dombrowski's more recent and nuanced *Babies and Beasts:*

The Argument from Marginal Cases (Chicago: University of Illinois Press, 1997). I have made a fuller argument against the "performance" account of human personhood in "What Is It Like to Be Bats Or Brains? Similarities and Differences Between Humans and Other Animals," *Modern Schoolman* 76 (November 1998).

NOTES TO CHAPTER FIVE

1. Immanuel Kant, *Fundamental Principles of the Metaphysics of Morals* (1785), trans. T. K. Abbott, in *Kant's Theory of Ethics*, Vol. 4 (London: Longmans, Green, and Co., 1990).
2. John Stuart Mill, *Utilitarianism*, in *Collected Works*, Vol. 10 (Toronto: University of Toronto Press, 1969).
3. *Summa Theologiae*, First Part, Question 5, Article 3, Reply to the second point. The translation is my own.
4. Several years ago I proposed a team-taught graduate seminar to Dr. Joseph Callahan, an adjunct professor of psychiatry at Saint Louis University. The title I proposed was "The Philosophical Foundations of Psychoanalysis." Callahan paused and said, "Why not 'The Psychoanalytic Foundations of Philosophy'?" He was right. We presume that philosophical models of knowledge dominate the methods of other disciplines. We often fail to see, however, how the domains of other disciplines, especially psychology, influence even the approach we might take to philosophy. Quite probably, neither Kant nor Nietzsche *could* have thought the way the other did.

   In my own experience, I noted as a graduate student in the 1970s that my interests at Washington University in Saint Louis were considered "quaint" or "romantic" by most of my teachers. I was interested in the human mind, in freedom, in death, in the exercise of power. Nietzsche was considered an impossibility for consideration; Hegel, barely. One of my logician teachers said that Hegel, Spinoza, or Kierkegaard might be considered, at best, poets. Then I understood. The strange fascination that this logician-professor exhibited for Quine was just that: a poetic, affective attachment—much like my own for the continental existentialists. What early childhood and infancy disciplines, I thought, could have led him to be so given to measurement, control, prediction, tidiness, and accuracy?
5. Carol Gilligan, *In A Different Voice: Psychological Theory and Woman's Development* (Cambridge, Mass.: Harvard University Press, 1982). There is a library of discussion and dispute over Gilligan's work. Some critics accuse her of dangerously reintroducing caricatures of "masculine" and "feminine" ways of thinking; others accuse her of elevating "an ethics of care"—a term wholly absent from Kant and Mill—to an unwarranted height. I think that Gilligan's truly significant work suffers from "either-or" forced dualisms

over gender as well as care-versus-justice. Rita C. Manning's *Speaking from the Heart: A Feminist Perspective on Ethics* (Lanham, Md.: Rowman & Littlefield, 1992) is a good survey of recent theories and issues. Like the work of Nel Noddings, Manning's is an ethics of care that stresses the interconnectedness of life, a contextual use of reason, a unity of theory and practice, and an experiential rejection of dualisms.

Alison M. Jaggar in *Feminist Politics and Human Nature* (Totowa, N.J.: Rowman & Allanheld, 1983) offers a range of approaches within feminist theory itself. Although Jaggar's work is directly concerned with social theory, it is suggestive in application to ethics. Among the considerable diversity in this relatively new area of research and theory, the most imaginative and, for some, abusive, work has been done by Mary Daly—for example, in *Gyn-Ecology: The Metaethics of Radical Feminism* (Boston: Beacon Press, 1978). For a good general introductory account of the feminist perspective, see Margaret Farley's "Feminism and Universal Morality," in *Prospects for a Common Morality*, ed. Gene Outka and John P. Reeder, Jr. (Princeton, N.J.: Princeton University Press, 1993). This entire collection (to which I refer in the context of other discussions), is excellent. Finally, Seyla Benhabib in *Situating the Self: Gender, Community and Postmodernism in Contemporary Ethics* (New York: Routledge, 1992) excels as a capacious and powerful interpreter of perspective in ethical discourse. Benhabib has a large historical range and a critical appreciation of contemporary debates; she proposes a universalism that is truly dialogical and open to diversity.

6. The debate over cognitivism versus noncognitivism is in many ways a debate over which internal factor dominates interest in ethical discussion. The noncognitivist most often will settle on the internal experience of intuition or feeling or emotion as the determinant of right and wrong. The cognitivist—among whom we would number Kant—emphasizes knowledge factors in ethical experience. Even here, there is a lurking forced dualism, resisting the integrated experience of an embodied person, insisting on the isolated cognitive or affective dimension as supreme, rather than the person herself.

7. Citations in this section are from Kant's *Fundamental Principles of the Metaphysics of Morals* (1785), in *Kant's Theory of Ethics*, Vol. 4, trans. T. K. Abbott (London: Longmans, Green, 1990), 9–20 *passim*.

Suggesting where to begin one's examination of Kantian ethics is hopelessly difficult, especially in view of the different kinds of reader one might have. For the general reader and college undergraduates, Roger Sullivan's *An Introduction to Kant's Ethics* (New York: Cambridge University Press, 1994) is an accessible and recent entry. It is valuable for its somewhat perspectival approach from the stance of political theory, as well as its attention to Kant's life and general philosophy. Sullivan's *Kant's Moral Theory*

(New York: Cambridge University Press, 1989) is more advanced, pene-trating, and rewarding. Another possible starting point might be *The Cambridge Companion to Kant*, edited by Paul Guyer (New York: Cambridge University Press, 1992). Guyer's introduction, Frederick C. Beiser's "Kant's Intellectual Development," and Schneewind's overview of Kant's moral philosophy are especially valuable. The treatment of Kant in histories of philosophy is best, I believe, in the straightforward Copleston series and the more demanding but utterly faithful work by James Collins in *A History of Modern European Philosophy* (Milwaukee, Wisc.: Bruce Publishing, 1954). L. W. Beck's *Commentary on Kant's Critique of Practical Reason* (Chicago: University of Chicago Press, 1960) is a valuable companion to Kant's ethics, although Rawls' study of the "Kantian constructivism" and Kantian social contract theory might be more satisfying and challenging. Kant also haunts the work of Alan Donagan, Robert Nozick, and Alan Gewirth. Another interesting approach would be to read Gilligan's *In a Different Voice* as a quarrel with Kant through his influence on Rawls, as well as Lawrence Kohlberg's *The Philosophy of Moral Development* (San Francisco: Harper and Row, 1981). Alan Donagan's *The Theory of Morality* (Chicago: University of Chicago Press, 1977) offers a critical and expanded Kantianism, emphasizing the dignity of the rational moral agent and its implications for the killing of persons.

More recently, G. Felicitas Munzel in *Kant's Conception of Moral Character: The Critical Link of Morality, Anthropology, and Reflective Judgement* (Chicago: University of Chicago Press, 1999) and Nancy Sherman's *Making a Necessity of Virtue: Aristotle and Kant on Virtue* (New York: Cambridge University Press, 1997) present astute interpretations of Kant that challenge the presumed account I offer in this chapter. Munzel and Sherman reveal the connections between Kant's moral theory and virtue, as well as anthropology.

8. This is not to deny that there are a host of "internal" relativisms, such as those mentioned earlier. My mood, feeling, emotion, ego, intuition, or sentiment could serve as my wholly internal criterion for what is right or wrong. Or I could simply choose to be internally skeptical about anything moral. Or I could negate morality as being personally meaningless for me. Or I could embrace a posture of cynicism. These positions are all relativisms with an internal twist.

By the way, my use of "internal and external turns" is somewhat different than that in David Brink's *Moral Realism and the Foundation of Ethics* (New York: Cambridge University Press, 1989), although I do appreciate his emphasis on the objective and "external" world in ethical reflection:

> Some think that internalism is the correct way to represent the practical character of morality and, therefore, that the practical character of morality tells

against moral realism. But moral realism is perfectly compatible with the practical character of morality. This is because externalism, rather than internalism, is the appropriate way to represent the practical or action-guiding character of morality. The rationality and motivational force of moral considerations depend, as the externalist claims, not simply on the concept of morality but (also) on the content of morality, facts about agents, and a substantive theory of reasons for action" (79–80).

With this, I wholly concur.

9. Although there is a *Cambridge Companion to Mill* edited by John Skorupski (New York: Cambridge University Press, 1998), the volume *Consequentialism and Its Critics*, edited by Samuel Scheffler (New York: Oxford University Press, 1988), may be a better place to witness the considerable diversity of positions and debate within utilitarianism. Because it focuses on the consequences aspect of an ethical act, moreover, it is more relevant to the comparisons I raise in the present discussion. Far more interesting are the contrasting evaluations of J. J. C. Smart (pro) and Bernard Williams (con) in *Utilitarianism: For and Against* (London: Cambridge University Press, 1973). Williams is especially crisp, as well as curt: "Any kind of utilitarianism is by definition consequentialist, but 'consequentialism' is the broader term, and in my use . . . utilitarianism is *one sort* of consequentialism which is specially concerned with happiness . . ." (79). Williams ends with this: "The important issues that utilitarianism raises should be discussed in contexts more rewarding than that of utilitarianism itself. The day cannot be too far off in which we hear no more of it" (150). Robin Barrow, in *Utilitarianism: A Contemporary Statement* (Brookfield, Vt.: Edward Elgar, 1991), begs to differ with that last statement of Williams.

10. This passage, as well as the following texts and redactions, are known famously from *Utilitarianism*. I have used the *Collected Works*, Vol. 10 (Toronto: University of Toronto Press, Routledge and Kegan Paul, 1969), Chapter 2, *passim*, especially 209–26.

    The whole issue of fulfillments and quality of life is taken up in a recent work sponsored by the World Institute for Development Economics Research. *Quality of Life*, edited by Martha Nussbaum (professor of philosophy and literature at Brown) and Amartya Sen (professor of philosophy and economics at Harvard) (Oxford: Clarendon Press, 1993), is a spotty but quite valuable collection of essays that probe the concrete national and international implications of moral positions and commitments. The section on traditions, relativism, and objectivity and the section on gender are particularly strong in the context of the full dimensions of moral action.

11. Vernon J. Bourke's *Ethics*, 2nd ed. (New York: Macmillan Co., 1966), remains an important source for anyone who is interested in Aquinas' approach. Bourke's selection of texts from Aquinas is particularly helpful in

locating strategic treatments of various topics, such as conscience and the constituents of a moral act. John Finnis' *Fundamentals of Ethics* (Washington D.C.: Georgetown University Press, 1983) and *Natural Law and Natural Rights* (Oxford: Clarendon, 1982) are equally valuable. Germain Grisez (who has published a massive presentation of Thomistic moral theology) has collaborated with Russell Shaw on *Beyond the New Morality* (Notre Dame, Ind.: Notre Dame University Press, 1980)—a defense of objectivity in ethics. Ralph McInerny's *Aquinas on Human Action: A Theory of Practice* (Washington, D.C.: Catholic University of America Press, 1992) is a closely reasoned and highly textual presentation of Thomistic ethical foundations. Henry Veatch's long-running defense of ethics grounded in human nature is aptly summed up in *Swimming Against the Current in Contemporary Philosophy* (Washington D.C.: Catholic University Press, 1990). George Klubertanz's *Habits and Virtues* (New York: Appleton-Century-Crofts, 1965) and the earlier *Philosophy of Human Nature* (New York: Appleton-Century-Crofts, 1953) are uncommonly fine presentations of Thomistic theory. A more recent treatment of virtues from the Thomistic tradition is Jean Porter's *The Recovery of Virtue* (Louisville, Ky.: Westminster Press, 1990). The ethical works of Jacques Maritain and John Courtney Murray's *We Hold These Truths* (New York: Sheed and Ward, 1960) are in the tradition of "intrinsicism." Most recently, Anthony Lisska offers a capacious account in Aquinas' *Theory of Natural Law: An Analytic Reconstruction* (Oxford: Clarendon Press, 1996).

William Luijpen's *Phenomenology of Natural Law* (Pittsburgh: Duquesne University Press, 1967) was one of the early attempts to integrate Thomism with 20th-century European phenomenology—a strategy later undertaken in the philosophical writings of Pope John Paul II. Although I have found both efforts attractive and helpful, Herbert Spiegelburg, the grand master of phenomenology, personally assured me that such attempts were not very successful from a phenomenologist's point of view. Some Thomists have expressed similar reservations.

If one wishes to examine a philosopher who understands the Thomistic and natural law traditions as well as debates within moral theology, one might explore Garth Hallett's *Reason and Right* (Notre Dame, Ind.: University of Notre Dame Press, 1984) and *Christian Moral Reasoning: An Analytic Guide* (Notre Dame, Ind.: University of Notre Dame Press, 1983). Hallett's work, which often is demanding and densely written and shows the influence of his extensive studies on Wittgenstein, presents a strong critique of essentialism and an impressive range of contemporary contributors.

Finally, one cannot afford to miss the contributions of Norman Kretzmann and Eleonore Stump. They are the editors of the *Cambridge Companion to Aquinas* (New York: Cambridge University Press, 1993), whose essay on

ethics is by Ralph McInerny. Stump also is the co-editor, with Scott Mac-
Donald, of *Aquinas' Moral Theory: Essays in Honor of Norman Kretzmann* (Ithaca,
N.Y.: Cornell University Press, 1999).

12. *S.T.* I, Q5, Art. 3, Response.

13. "You could call something perfect, in the sense of goodness, if there is
nothing lacking in its own appropriate form of being. Now anything that
exists has to exist as some kind of being, with its defined or determinate
form, with its own constitutive elements and capacities. Thus, for something to be realized (perfect) and good, it must have its own form with its
own requirements and capacities" (*S.T.* I, Q5, Art.5, Response, second sentence). I have developed this notion of intrinsic good more fully in "Intrinsic Values, Persons and Stewardship," in *The Challenge of Global Stewardship*,
ed. Maura Ryan and Todd Whitmore (Notre Dame, Ind.: University of
Notre Dame Press, 1977), 67–81.

14. John Kleinig in *Valuing Life* (Princeton, N.J.: Princeton University Press,
1991) presents an instructive range of the meanings of *good*, including the
intrinsic notion I have examined. In addition to the contributions of
Habermas and the critical theory school, the work of Bernstein and Schrag,
and the writings of Charles Taylor, one can find an alternative approach in
the works of the late John Macmurray, who bridges philosophical anthropology and ethics. "The Crisis of the Personal" is his lead chapter in *The Self
As Agent* (New York: Humanities Press, 1978 [1957]). Macmurray's *Persons in
Relation* (London: Faber and Faber, 1935) and *Freedom in the Modern World*
(New York: Harper and Row, 1961), like other works of his that once were
out of print, are attracting a resurgence of interest.

15. Timothy McVeigh, "An Essay on Hypocrisy," *Media Bypass Magazine*, June
1998.

16. Mill, *On Liberty* (introduction to any edition). See *Collected Works*, Vol. 10
(Toronto: University of Toronto Press, 1969). A collection of essays on
Autonomy, The Inner Citadel, edited by John Christman (New York: Oxford
University Press, 1989) presents contrasting approaches from Kantian and
Mill perspectives, although the notion of intrinsic value is not offered as a
constraint on liberty.

NOTES TO CHAPTER SIX

1. Charles Taylor, "Explanation and Practical Reason," in *The Quality of Life*,
ed. Martha Nussbaum and Amartya Sen (Oxford: Clarendon Press, 1993).
208.

2. Robert Hughes, *The Culture of Complaint: The Fraying of America* (New York:
Oxford University Press, 1993). This book itself is a complaint—but an
often delightful and challenging one. Hughes' basic thrust is to unmask the

moral selectivity and snobbish superiority of the right and the left, of extreme feminists and extreme evangelicals, of academics as well as politicians. This book is snappier and broader than other published "complaints" such as Dinesh D'Souza's *Illiberal Education* (New York: Free Press, 1991), Charles Sykes' *A Nation of Victims* (New York: Saint Martin's Press, 1993), and Thomas Sowell's *Inside American Education* (New York: Free Press, 1992).

3. Vaclav Havel, "The End of the Modern Era," *New York Times*, op-ed page, March 1, 1992.

4. Calvin Schrag, whose model of experience as a dynamic field I discussed earlier, offers an integrated understanding of human reason—"transversal" reason—as the bridge between the seemingly disparate realms of subjectivity and nature. In *The Resources of Rationality: A Response to the Post-Modern Challenge* (Bloomington: Indiana University Press, 1992), he presents a chastened reason—having learned from the postmodern critique of enlightenment, traveled through Husserl's "crisis" of modern thought, followed Ricoeur through his hermeneutics of suspicion and recovery, and accompanied Habermas in his discourse over modernity.

Schrag is well aware of the contemporary assault on "despised logos" mounted by Rorty, Derrida, Lyotard, Foucault, and others who follow the charting of Nietzsche and Heidegger into the land of postmodernity. Schrag appreciates the unmasking of the stratagems of power and desire lurking behind the clear and distinct lines of rationality. He also is unafraid of plurality and indeterminacy, for he proposes a critical and discerning rationality as our guide. This rationality—much like our notion of reflexive consciousness as embodied—yields a "discernment" that is intrinsically communal, linguistic, and self-challenging. Such is the stuff of human reason's embeddedness in self-narrative and life-world. Discernment is the activity of a *human* reason, defined by the journey of speakers and actors lodged in a dense world of talk, perception, and action. It is a reason that is not confined to any specific discourse or form of knowledge but operative *between* forms of knowledge. It is an integrative mapping of other maps.

The theory of "embodied self-consciousness" shares this notion of human rationality—not an isolated sphere of the disembodied experiencer or pure subject but an integrated act of an integrated person.

5. See discussion in Chapter 7 of Freud's *Civilization and Its Discontents*, trans. James Strachey (New York: Norton, 1961), 70–80. "His aggressiveness is introjected, internalized; it is, in point of fact, sent back to where it came from—that is, it is directed towards his own ego. There it is taken over by a portion of the ego, which sets itself over against the rest of the ego as super-ego, and which now, in the form of '*conscience,*' is ready to put into action against the ego the same harsh aggressiveness that the ego would have liked to satisfy upon other, extraneous individuals. The tension between

the harsh super-ego and the ego that is subjected to it, is called by us the sense of guilt" (70).

In a splendid irony, Bernard Lonergan reflects on Freud's conscience: "When Freud decided eventually to publish his *Traumdeutung* [*Interpretation of Dreams*], he was overcoming emotions and sentiments and following what he considered the only intelligent and reasonable course of action; and such following is what we mean by obeying moral conscience." *Insight: A Study of Human Understanding* (New York: Philosophical Library, 1958), 600.

6. Cf. *Summa Theologica*, Ia, lxxix, 13, and *Quodlibet*, III, 27.

7. Mary Midgley, in *Can't We Make Moral Judgements?* (New York: Saint Martin's Press, 1991), offers a somewhat different and larger context for the word "judgment." Whereas I use "moral judgment" as the defining equivalent to "conscience"—wherein I am judging the rightness or wrongness of an act before me—Midgley uses the more common association of making "moral judgments" about behaviors, especially those of others. Her approach actually is an extended discussion of whether we can overcome pure emotivism or relativism in ethics. She helpfully points out, however, some of the distortions in the use of "moral judgment" in this way: too often applied only to others, too often unfavorable and uncharitable, too often about a past act, and too often from a detached position (30). With such associations—so exclusive of all the internal dimensions—no wonder "making judgments" has such a bad taste.

8. Lawrence Kohlberg, in *The Philosophy of Moral Development: Moral Stages and the Idea of Justice* (New York: Harper and Row, 1981), is the most visible and influential proponent of moral stages—six of them, over three levels of preconventional, conventional, and postconventional moral development. Moral development passes through responsiveness to punishment, self-interest, living up to others' expectations, duty, rights and social contract, and finally universal ethical principles. This approach is strongly contested in the work of Carol Gilligan and the earlier work of Nel Noddings, *Caring: A Feminine Approach to Ethics and Moral Education* (Berkeley: University of California Press, 1978).

9. This false separation of the "internal" from the "external" was magisterially revealed by Hegel. Not surprisingly, then, one of the preeminent Hegel scholars attempted to unmask the spurious dichotomy between individuality (the internal and the subjective) and social reality. Charles Taylor, whose masterful work dealt with "sources" of the self rather than the "end" of it, proposes in *The Ethics of Authenticity* that modernity has reached a "malaise" by following a constricting map of the human person.

Individualism, in our present cultural crisis, poses as enthroned subjectivity, as subjectivism. Its hallmark is a relativism that many people, Taylor contends, unquestioningly accept. He also thinks such relativism is wrongheaded, in that it undercuts the ideal of authenticity on which it is based. It erodes the capacities of human intelligence to which it appeals. It dissolves the freedom in the name of which individualism is defended. As Taylor points out, once you see the cultural and historical forces behind the notion of authenticity, it cannot even be what it is, if it is reduced to a crude subjectivist relativism (29).

The cultural ideal of authenticity requires, however, that we ask ourselves what conditions might fulfill it. If we investigate the matter, we surely will find the dialogical conditions of language, intersubjectivity, and community ever present. There also is an inescapable but covert appeal to rational intelligibility underwriting our insistence on personal ideals and significance. It gives the content of "self-choice" whatever coherence it may have. Even more, there can be no nontrivial answer to personal significance that excludes the external factors of history, society, nature, or solidarity. "Authenticity is not the enemy of demands that emanate from beyond the self; it supposes such demands" (41).

Similarly, the very affirmation of uniqueness and difference requires an immediate recognition of the commonality between all beings that claim such uniqueness. Claims for authenticity are grounded not in sheer difference or individuality in themselves but in the commonly shared capacities of reason, or love, or memory, or dialogical recognition that constitute the valorization of our uniqueness.

Without the complementary mappings of intelligence, community, and language, authenticity careens into mere narcissism and atomism, turning from theories of nihilism and untrammeled power to culturally legitimized self-infatuation. A contentless "choice" without social or intelligible horizons is all that is left for human self-guidance and self-understanding.

Yet a probing of the ideal of authenticity not only reveals conditions that are opposed to its contemporary deviance; it yields possibilities for common ground and interest. "What we ought to be doing is fighting over the meaning of authenticity, and from the standpoint developed here, we ought to be trying to persuade people that self-fulfillment, so far from excluding unconditional relationships and moral demands beyond the self, actually requires these in some form. The struggle ought not to be *over* authenticity, for or against, but *about* it, defining its proper meaning. We ought to be trying to lift the culture back up, closer to its motivating ideal" (73). Unfortunately, rather than closely examining the value of the authenticity ideal, rather than establishing in reason what such an ideal involves, rather than admitting that such an ideal makes a difference in practice, discourse has hardened into polar ideologies. Critics of wild (but one-sided) subjectivism offer anathemas. Proponents offer apologetics.

The only solution to the fragmentation of the academy, the body politic, and the individual body, Taylor proposes, is a dialectical understanding of the embodied human person, endowed with a rational capacity that is neither ahistorical nor merely instrumental but fully dialogical, communal, and historically enfleshed. Such has been the goal of Charles Taylor's labors, from his luminous study of Hegel to his *Sources of the Self*. Steeped in the history of philosophy, Taylor is not so grand as to be convinced that it has ended. (I have also made these observations, as well as those on Schrag and Michael McCarthy, in a feature review in the *Modern Schoolman* in 1993.)

10. From Hume's assertion that our revulsion to or condemnation of murder was a matter of feeling rather than reason in his *Treatise on Human Nature* to the contemporary trump card in all ethical debates, "It's an emotional issue," the full range of argument over subjectivism, emotivism, and relativisms of other sort merits—and has received—many extended treatments. C. L Stevenson's *Ethics and Language* (New Haven, Conn.: Yale University Press, 1944); A. J. Ayer's *Language, Truth and Logic* (London: Gollancz, 1936), especially Chapter 6; J. L. Mackie's *Ethics: Inventing Right and Wrong* (Harmondsworth, England: Penguin, 1977), and Stevenson's *Facts and Values* (New Haven, Conn.: Yale University Press, 1963), as well as other influential "philosophical" academic treatments, do not carry as much weight as they once did; a day of talk shows and editorial columns is enough to convince, however, that a combined form of utilitarianism, emotivism, and relativism reigns supreme in our cultural consciousness.

11. This is not to deny that there is a startling unity and universality across ages and cultures concerning many foundational ethical principles. In fact there is more agreement on "The Golden Rule" than in the history of mathematics or the conclusions of natural science.

Hinduism: "This is the sum of duty: Do nothing to others which would cause you pain if done to you" (*Mahabharata* 5, 1517).

Buddhism: "Hurt not others in ways that you yourself would find harmful" (*Udana-Varga* 5, 18).

Confucianism: "Is there one maxim which ought to be acted upon throughout one's life? Surely it is the maxim of loving-kindness: Do not do to others what you would not have them do to you" (*Analects* 15, 23).

Taoism: "Regard your neighbor's gain as your own gain, and your neighbor's loss as your own loss" (*Tai Shang Kan Ying*).

Zoroastrianism: "That nature alone is good which refrains from doing to another whatever is not good for its own self" (*Dadistan-i-Dinik*, 94, 5).

Judaism: "What is hateful to you, do not do to your fellow men and women. That is the entire Law: All the rest is commentary" (*Talmud, Shabbat*, 3).

Christianity: "Treat others the way you want them to treat you. This is the Law and the Prophets" (Mt. 7:12).

Islam: "No one of you is a believer until he desires for his brothers that which he desires for himself" (*Hadith*).

Baha'i Faith: "He should not wish for others that which he does not wish for himself" (*Gleanings*).

C. S. Lewis' "Tao of Ethics" in his little polemic *The Abolition of Man* (New York: Macmillan, 1947) collects a wide-ranging series of ethical principles from the religions of the world in a variety of topics.

12. Michael McCarthy provides just this kind of investigation into the objectively required conditions for human "insight" in *The Crisis of Philosophy* (Albany: State University of New York Press, 1990). Using the cognitively integrative method of Bernard Lonergan's *Insight* and his own Aristotelian sensibilities, McCarthy reviews the historical conditions of modern philosophy that have led to the present cul-de-sac for disembodied rationality. The book has breathtaking range—encountering phenomenology, linguistic analysis, and logical positivism as well as recent contemporaries such as Rorty.

Like Calvin Schrag, McCarthy resists the polarizing tendencies of physicalists who relocate human reason in nature and historicists who reduce it to culture. McCarthy agrees that there is a splintering devastation in the late-modern Cartesian and Kantian enterprises—but only because of a fundamental disintegration fated from the start. Thus, rather than advise, with Rorty, an abandonment of the human quest for cognitive integration, McCarthy turns to Lonergan for a new integrative strategy. "The classical tradition was not wrong to insist on something substantial and common to human nature and cognitive activity, but it failed to appreciate how that common ground was the basis for continuous historical development" (xix). The universal and invariant structure to human cognition—of which all other cognitive enterprises are instantiations—is not opposed to historical change at all. It is the condition of its possibility and meaning.

McCarthy, then, has no fear of foundations or starting points. He simply mistrusts those that are located in something other than the intentional historical subject called the human person.

McCarthy's *cognitive integration* is centered in the notion of the "intentional subject," the human reality of being a conscious subject of experience—not as a transcendental subject, not as a disembodied mind, but as an ontologically unified, embodied reality that is capable of taking possession of its own experience. "Philosophy is the flowering of the individual's intentional consciousness in its coming to know and take possession of itself" (233). Every philosophical enterprise entails the exercise of our "experiential consciousness," our prereflexive, nonintentional awareness of ourselves and our intentional acts. This is not introspection or analysis; it is our very capacity of intending. This is not some self who, like Hume, goes out hoping to spot itself. It is the condition for the going, the hoping, and the spotting.

"In the process of personal appropriation, intentional subjects discover the concrete, experientially conscious conditions of their continuing existences as knowers. These foundational conditions are the source and principle of every cognitive achievement and revision; they are not causal products of cultural advance and development but the prior grounds of their possibility. They exist, generally unacknowledged, at the very center of who we are as human persons" (257).

13. There is a short biography of Byers Naude, with a series of testimonials, in Peter Randall, ed., *Not Without Honour* (Johannesburg: Raven Press, 1982). In court testimony, Naude noted, "In order to determine the causes of injustice, a person must not only have the outward individual facts of the matter, but as a Christian you are called to identify yourself in heart and soul, to live in, to think in, and to feel in the hearts, in the consciousness, the feelings, of the person or the persons who feel themselves aggrieved." This is a powerful integration of the external and internal dimensions of conscience.

14. From the viewpoint of a psychologist with strong anthropological themes, Jerome Bruner's *Acts of Meaning* (Cambridge, Mass.: Harvard University Press, 1990) makes a powerful case for the cultural and social constitution of the self as well as the moral point of view. Bruner never omits the strategic fact of human "capacity," "readiness," or "predisposition" that makes possible meaning, symbol, and culture itself. "While we have an 'innate' and primitive predisposition to narrative organization that allows us quickly and easily to comprehend and use it, the culture soon equips us with new powers of narration through its tool kit and through the traditions of telling and interpreting in which we soon come to participate" (80).

15. The Gandhi passage is from Louis Fischer's anthology, *The Essential Gandhi* (New York: Vintage, 1963), 200.

16. King's "Letter from a Birmingham Jail" appears in *Why We Can't Wait* (New York: Harper, 1963), 77–100. The reference to Aquinas appears on page 85.

17. A powerful examination of the dynamics of conscience appears in a little-known biography, Gordon Zahn, *In Solitary Witness: The Life and Death of Franz Jägerstätter* (Collegeville, Minn.: Liturgical Press, 1964). In his "prison statement," Jägerstätter writes: "For what purpose, then, did God endow all men with reason and free will if, despite this, we have to render blind obedience [to Hitler]; or if, as so many also say, the individual is not qualified to judge whether this war started by Germany is just or unjust?" (233).

18. Marilyn French's *The War Against Women* (New York: Ballantine, 1992) is just one of the more recent surveys of the ways women are treated as less than human while the data are suppressed. Although some readers claim that French's book is tendentious and wildly conspiracy-minded, the outrages she catalogues are largely undeniable. She indicts religious institutions and states. She discusses genital mutilation, female infanticide, the cruelties of Iran's secret police, and the general "War Against Women's Personhood." Unfortunately, there is absolutely no philosophical justification for her outrage. Without a theory of fundamental personal dignity, every crime she lists is justifiable.

19. Camus' *The Fall* (New York: Vintage, 1956), *The Plague* (New York: Vintage, 1991), and *The Stranger* (New York: Vintage, 1989) are uncommonly brilliant moral narratives that confront the issue of evil more directly and profoundly than most nonfiction ethics treatises. He apparently holds little respect as a philosopher, although his treatments of suicide in *The Myth of Sisyphus* (New York: Vintage, 1991) and of political murder in *The Rebel* (New York: Vintage, 1991) are brilliant confrontations with issues of life and death. Subject as academia is to the laws of the market, I believe his impact will be felt once again—not for its novelty but for its passion.

20. Camus, *The Fall*,. 84, 101, and *passim*.

21. *Ibid.*, 142.

22. *Ibid.*, 44.

23. *Ibid.*, 68.

24. *Ibid.*, 143.

25. All quotations are from *Crimes and Misdemeanors*, directed by Woody Allen (a Jack Rollins and Charles Jaffe Production, Orion Films). In many ways, this film is a contemporary reformulation of Plato's "Ring of Gyges" in the first book of *The Republic*.

NOTES TO CHAPTER SEVEN

1. Friedrich Nietzsche, *The Philosophy of Nietzsche*, ed. Geoffrey Clive (New York: Mentor, 1965), 425 (*Twilight of the Idols*).

2. *Rwanda: Death, Despair and Defiance* (London: African Rights, 1995), 639.

3. Peter Singer, *Rethinking Life and Death* (New York: St. Martin's Press, 1995), 255.

4. Erich H. Loewy, "Harming, Healing, and Euthanasia," in *Regulating How We Die*, ed. Linda Emanuel (Cambridge, Mass.: Harvard University Press, 1998), 66.

5. Nietzsche, *Human, All Too Human*, 372. His reference to "degenerate life" might apply to an 1981 incident. Peter Singer recounts the famous trial of a doctor who refused to provide treatment and accelerated the death of a

Down's syndrome baby. "The most eminent of all the medical practitioners in court, however, was Sir Douglas Black, President of the Royal College of Physicians, who told the jury he thought it 'would be ethical to put a rejected child upon a course of management that would end in its death. . . . I say that it is ethical that a child suffering from Down's syndrome . . . should not survive.'" *Rethinking Life and Death*, 122–23.

6. The background and statement of Yousef appears in "Mastermind Gets Life for Bombing of Trade Center," *New York Times*, January 9, 1998, A1, A15.

Stephen Segaller's *Invisible Armies: Terrorism into the 1990s* (New York: Harcourt Brace and Jovanovich, 1987) and Walter Reich's *Origins of Terrorism: Psychologies, Ideologies, Theologies, States of Mind* (New York: Cambridge, 1990) offer fuller treatments of the logic of terror. See also Human Rights Watch, *Slaughter Among Neighbors* (New Haven, Conn.: Yale University Press, 1995), for treatments of incidents in Israel, India, Kenya, Sri Lanka.

If one fails to comprehend the claims of Arab extremists, one might consider reading about the Jewish surgical bombing of Lebanon in "Dark With Blood," *Time*, April 29, 1996, 53–59: "The devastation was sickening, a carnage of incinerated corpses, body parts and blood. 'I couldn't count the bodies,' said Swedish U.N. Captain Mikael Lindwass at the compound right after the attack. 'There were babies without heads. There were people without arms or legs.'" Of the Lebanon bombing, Jewish writer Ari Shavit later wrote, "The yawning gap between the unlimited sacrosanct importance we attribute to our own lives and the very limited sacred character we attribute to the lives of others allowed us to kill them. . . . Arrogance. Egocentricism of the strong. A penchant to blur the distinction between good and bad, the allowed and the forbidden." "How Easily We Killed Them," *New York Times*, May 27, 1996.

7. *Cf.* Barbara Crossette, "Civilians Will be in Harm's Way if Baghdad is Hit," *New York Times*, January 28, 1998, and Steven Lee Myers, "Whether to Bomb is the Easy Part," *New York Times*, February 1, 1998. The effects of sanctions and periodic bombings on Iraq are catalogued in *Living Under Sanctions In Iraq: The Oil-For-Food Program and The Intellectual Embargo* (Philadelphia: American Friends Service Committee, 1999).

8. The statement is recounted by Henry Louis Gates—who, in discussing the cases of extremism mentioned here, calls for "A Liberalism of Heart and Spine," grounded in the conviction of our "shared humanity." *New York Times*, op-ed page, March 27, 1994.

9. *Ibid*. The "dehumanization" tactic is imaginatively portrayed in Sam Keen's *Faces of the Enemy: Reflections of the Hostile Imagination* (San Francisco: Harper and Row, 1986).

10. This final statement was made by Moshe Gross, of Brooklyn, quoted in "Where the Killer is a Hero," *U.S. News and World Report*, November 20, 1995, 74.

11. For a general introduction to the issues, Louis Pojman's reader, *Life And Death* (Boston: Jones and Bartlett, 1993), is serviceable, although it is weakened by the fact that its only "classical theorists" are Kant, Mill, and Hobbes. The topics range from suicide and abortion to war, capital punishment, animal rights, and starvation.

12. Lt. Col. Dave Grossman, *On Killing: The Psychological Cost of Learning to Kill in War and Society* (Boston: Little, Brown, 1995), 88–89. Richard Norman, in *Ethics of Killing and War* (New York: Cambridge University Press, 1995)—a "pacifistic" approach to the issue—expresses well the intuitive acknowledgement of some foundational betrayal in the act of killing: "I have argued in this book that the idea of the wrongness of taking a human life is not something which we can just take or leave. It is a deep feature of our structure of moral understanding, grounded in our most basic human responses. As such it has an objective validity, and this remains true however much people may go against it is practice, and whatever further claims they may make about possible reasons for overriding it" (251). For a range of discussions about the "absolute" nature of the no-killing standard offered here, Joram Graf Haber, ed., *Ablolutism and Its Consequentialist Critics* (Lanham, Md.: Rowman and Littlefield, 1994), is worth examining.

13. The absence of this insight, for example, characterizes one of the finer treatments—Tom L. Beauchamp and James F. Childress, *Principles of Biomedical Ethics*, 3rd ed. (New York: Oxford University Press, 1989). This book is an outstanding presentation of cases, argued against the background of deontological and consequential ethics. There is even a final treatment of virtue and heroic ethics. Yet there is no extended discussion of the criteria we might use to determine a human person or the implications of an intrinsic theory of human dignity.

14. Two of the more powerful accounts of the Rwanda tragedy appear in *The Tablet*, June 18, 1994, and Alex Shoumatoff's "Flight from Death," *The New Yorker*, June 20, 1994, 44–55; the first quotation is from page 53. The four subsequent testimonials are from the massive study *Rwanda: Death, Despair and Defiance* (London: African Rights, 1995), 996, 998, 1002, 799. The last quotation of the set is from Gerard Prunier's *The Rwanda Crisis: History of a Genocide* (New York: Columbia University Press, 1995), 247.

For four contrasting and somewhat "classical" philosophical approaches to war, W. B. Gallie's collection, *Philosophers of Peace and War: Kant, Clausewitz, Marx, Engels and Tolstoy* (Cambridge: Cambridge University Press, 1978), is valuable. Howard P. Kainz has a wide-ranging collection in *Philosophical Perspectives on Peace: An Anthology of Classical and Modern Sources* (Athens, Ohio:

Ohio University Press, 1987). Paul Ramsey's *The Just War: Force and Political Responsibility* (New York: Scribner, Littlefield Adams, 1968) and Michael Walzer's *Just and Unjust Wars: A Moral Argument with Historical Illustrations* (New York: Basic Books, 1977) are standard works. James Turner Johnson and John Kelsay, eds., *Cross, Crescent, and Sword: The Justification and Limitation of War in Western and Islamic Tradition* (New York: Greenwood Press, 1990), reveals the range of justifications for violence across cultures and religions.

15. Thomas Nagel, "War and Massacre," in *International Ethics*, ed. C. R. Beitz et al. (Princeton, N.J.: Princeton University Press, 1985), 73.

16. In the episode "Total War" of the PBS series *People's Century* (aired June 1998), the mentality of defense and just retribution is harrowingly presented. A British midwife during the bombing of Plymouth remembers, "Yes, I thought that if they could do this to us, do it to children, we should do it to them. I know it wasn't a nurse's philosophy at all to feel like that, but that's the way I felt then. 'Do it to them.'" Hakudo Nagatomi, one of the Japanese who slaughtered Chinese, recounts his army's slogan: "The three Alls: 'Burn all, steal all, kill all.' That means if there were people, kill them, if there was a house, burn it, if there were cows or sheep, slaughter them. . . . I did many terrible things."

17. One wonders about, for example, the implication of George Will's position that "capital punishment is justified as a clear and controlled means for a nation to express feelings that are not only justified but are indispensable to civilization; feelings such as implacable rage about assaults on the social order." Stalin or French leftist supporters of Mao might take Will's justification a long way. A more rational treatment—albeit by someone who opposes capital punishment—is Hugo Adam Bedau's *Studies in the Morality, Law, and Politics of Capital Punishment* (Boston: Northeastern University Press, 1987). I also recommend Helen Prejean, C.S.J., *Dead Man Walking: An Eyewitness Account of the Death Penalty in the United States* (New York: Random House, 1993).

18. This is quite a different reading of personhood, consequently, than that in Mary Anne Warren's *Moral Status: Obligations to Persons and Other Living Things* (Oxford: Clarendon Press, 1977). Warren's notion of person and "moral status" is reduced to a human construction, rather than any biological or ontological reality. Her reading, moreover, of the early stages of human development and potentiality, as observed in other citations, is systematically opposite to the ones proposed herein. See especially Chapters 8 and 9. Kevin Doran, in *What Is a Person: The Concept and the Implications for Ethics* (Lewiston, N.Y.: Edwin Mellon Press, 1989), reviews variant renderings of personhood, offers the argument that the conceptus is a distinct living substance, and then applies it to the cases of *in vitro* fertilization and embryo transfer.

19. One of the most informative treatments of the early stages of human development is *When Did I Begin: Conception of the Human Individual in History, Philosophy and Science* (New York: Cambridge University Press, 1991) by Norman Ford—a moral philosopher who is quite conversant in embryology.
Even in the context of Aristotelian "soul" theory (the soul is the dynamic
unifying principle of a living being), Ford offers evidence that there is no
dynamic individual acting as a unity until the onset of the second week
after conception: the "primitive streak," the last stage at which identical
twins might be formed:

> This appears to be the stage of development when the cells of the epiblast first
> become organized through this primitive streak into one whole multicellular in-
> dividual living human being, possessing for the first time a body axis and bilat-
> eral symmetry. Its developing cells are now integrated and subordinated to form
> a single heterogeneous organic body that endures with its own ontological as
> well as biological identity through all its subsequent stages of growth and devel-
> opment. A new human individual begins once the matter of the epiblastic cells
> becomes one living body, informed or actuated by a human form, life-principle
> or soul that arises through the creative power of God. The appearance of one
> primitive streak signals that only one embryo proper and human individual has
> been formed and begun to exist. Prior to this stage it would be pointless to speak
> about the presence of a true human being in an ontological sense. A human indi-
> vidual could scarcely exist before a definite human body is formed. As men-
> tioned earlier, the formation of an ontological individual with a truly human na-
> ture and rational ensoulment must coincide (171–72).

Ford has the entire paragraph in emphasis. Although I put greater emphasis on the genetic coding of identity, I believe a thoughtful reflection
such as this must give pause to people who hold my position when we seek
to protect the life of any human being by political action. Such political
protection, by definition, must be based on evidence that is acceptable to
the people who are affected by the decision.

20. See Baruch Brody's *Abortion and the Sanctity of Human Life: A Philosophical View*
(Cambridge, Mass.: MIT Press, 1975). A strong challenge to any theory
holding that we are only our brains or our conscious acts appears in Eric T.
Olson, *The Human Animal: Personal Identity Without Psychology* (New York:
Oxford University Press, 1997), which takes seriously the fact that human
persons are animals. If the person John Kavanaugh is only his psychic
states, I am faced with the troubling conclusion that somewhere along the
line after the development of some organism (which was not me), upon becoming conscious I came into existence somehow attached to this strange
body. Olson's brilliant book shows the "cortical" Cartesianism of many
contemporary discussions, which always presume that we are brains, not
living, bodied beings endowed with psychic capacities.

21. Again opposed to the position offered here, Mary Ann Warren in "Abortion," in *A Companion to Ethics*, ed. Peter Singer (Cambridge: Blackwell, 1991), states, "Some philosophers argue that, although fetuses may not be persons, their potential to *become* persons gives them the same basic moral rights. . . . If a fetus is a potential person, then so is an unfertilized human ovum, together with enough viable spermatozoa to achieve fertilization; yet few would seriously suggest that *these* living human entities should have full and moral status" (312). That her argument is seriously flawed is evident in her earlier discussion of "genetic humanity," where she must confront the actual humanity status of a conceived human. In this case, she has to resort to the question of whether humans are special anyway. In the citation above, the issue is not potential personhood. It is personhood with potential. No informed person thinks a sperm by itself is a potential person or is the same existentially as a conceived human. There is absolutely no evidence to support such a statement, unless one wishes to return to the medieval biological view that a sperm or an ovum is a little "homunculus."

Warren, whose article "The Personhood Argument in Favor of Abortion," *The Monist* 57, no. 1 (1973), stirred many responses because it seemed to justify infanticide, offered a chilling postscript in a later edition of the article in Louis Pojman, *Life and Death: A Reader in Moral Problems* (Boston: Jones and Bartlett, 1993):

> Now, if I am right in holding that it is only people who have a full-fledged right to life, and who can be murdered, and if the criteria of personhood are as I have described them, then it obviously follows that killing a newborn infant isn't murder. It does *not* follow, however, that infanticide is permissible, for two reasons. In the first place, it would be wrong, at least in this country and in this period of history, and other things being equal, to kill a new-born infant, because even if its parents do not want it and would not suffer from its destruction, there are other people who would like to have it, and would, in all probability, be deprived of a great deal of pleasure by its destruction. Thus, infanticide is wrong for reasons analogous to those which make it wrong to wantonly destroy natural resources, or great works of art. . . .
>
> On the other hand, it follows from my argument that when an unwanted or defective infant is born into a society which cannot afford or is not willing to care for it, then its destruction is permissible. This conclusion will, no doubt, strike many people as heartless and immoral; but remember that the very existence of people who feel this way, and who are willing and able to provide care for unwanted infants, is reason enough to conclude that they should be preserved."

Many animal rights philosophers, such as Pluhar, associate "full personhood" with specific performance criteria, such as expressed conscious action and intent. Dan Dombrowski, who sympathizes with the animal rights theorists, presents an excellent summary of their debates in *Babies and Beasts: The Argument from Marginal Cases* (Urbana: University of Illinois Press, 1997). His efforts are not so much to degrade the moral status of the infant as to raise the moral status of other animals.

22. The dumpster story is from *New York Newsday*, February 3, 1993. The botched abortion story is from "Jury Hears Grisly Tale: Baby's Arm Severed During Abort Try," *Daily News*, January 30, 1993, 5, and "Abortion Doc Case Tough on Potential Jurors," *New York Newsday*, January 23, 1993, 18. The doctor was found guilty.

23. Sagan offered his position in popular interviews, Hentoff in his columns for *The Village Voice*, and Nathanson in videos—particularly *The Silent Scream*.

24. See the discussion in note 17 to this chapter for the primitive streak argument.

25. Ronald Dworkin in *Life's Dominion: An Argument about Abortion, Euthanasia, and Individual Freedom* (New York: Alfred A. Knopf, 1993) seems to contrast life's intrinsic value or "sacredness" with the issue of rights. Sacredness, for Dworkin (as opposed to the position taken in radical personalism) is essentially a religious concept and thereby separable from political life and legislation. He is quite sympathetic to the sacredness argument and, for this reason, likely to win considerable disapproval from anyone who does not wish the humanity status of the fetus to be raised. At the same time, he seems incapable of understanding the "pro-life" argument that unborn humans are indeed human and deserving of the law's protection. John Kleinig in *Valuing Life* (Princeton, N.J.: Princeton University Press, 1991) provides a valuable discussion of "potentiality" and "capacity" with a level nuance that is rare in contemporary debate. Kleinig's book is a careful treatment of "life" in all of its forms; he offers conclusions that are at variance with this work.

26. Not only was the biological evidence scanty; the guesswork was haphazard (brilliant as Aristotle and Aquinas may have been). In their ethical theories, the foundational principle of human dignity was often abandoned in the breech. Thus, overriding a solid theory of human nature, both were able to justify slavery and dangerously misread the place of women in the natural and political order. A biologistically weighted view of human sexuality stifled the personal dimensions that, in Aquinas' own theory, should have been equally important. Capital punishment, an issue convoluted even more drastically in Kant, is justified.

27. *Compassion in Dying v. State of Washington*, 79 F.3d 790, Ninth Circuit (1996). This decision, with its focus on "the liberty interest," has powerful echoes of Mill's words: "The only freedom which deserves the name is that of pursuing our own good in our own way, so long as we do not attempt to deprive others of their efforts to obtain it. Each is the proper

guardian of his own health, whether bodily or mental and spiritual." John Stuart Mill, *On Liberty* (New York: Penguin, 1988 [1859]). Although there is a powerful undercurrent of self–others dualism as well as a dangerous "exceptionalism"—for "barbarians," for example—Mill's work seems to be the reigning standard of political moral consciousness in the United States. *Cf.* pp. 71, 72.

28. Derek Humphry, *Final Exit* (Eugene, Ore.: Hemlock Society, 1991).

29. The story appeared in many publications. Quotations and data presented here are from the *New York Times Magazine*, November 24, 1991, 86, 88.

30. Martin S. Pernick, *The Black Stork* (New York: Oxford University Press, 1996), 21–23.

31. These questions are not far-fetched. "In an effort to end the sale of human organs by the country's poor, Egyptian doctors have announced a ban on all kidney transplants from living donors that are not done between relatives. . . . Private laboratories often act as brokerage houses, sending out recruiters to the slums of Cairo to entice prospective donors in for tissue tests. Kidneys sell for $10,000 to $15,000. Dr. Barsoum said he has even heard of auctions, with the organ going to the highest bidder." *New York Times*, January 23, 1992. The strongest presentation of the problem appears in Andrew Kimbrell's *The Human Body Shop: The Engineering and Marketing of Life* (San Francisco: Harper, 1993): "We can continue to adhere, in near religious fashion, to the centuries-old dogmas of mechanism and the market. We can continue to view our bodies as machines and commodities. We can continue to remake our bodies with surgery and genetic engineering. We can continue to manipulate the reproductive process by eliminating the birth of children with undesirable traits. We can continue to alter with drugs and genetic therapies those with 'abnormal' traits. We can continue to clone life-forms and human body parts. We can continue to permit the international sale of organs, the commercialization of fetal parts, the sale of sperm and eggs, and the patenting of animals and human genes and cells" (284). (He hopes not.)

32. Jack Kevorkian, *Prescription Medicine: The Goodness of Planned Death* (Buffalo: Prometheus Press, 1991).

33. Robert Jay Lifton, *The Nazi Doctors* (New York: Basic Books, 1986), 113. In the "Master Race" episode of the PBS series *People's Century*, Jurgen Kroger—a repentant executioner for Nazi death squads—recounts, "They said the Jews were an inferior race. One of them said to me, 'It's like having a rosebush and the rosebush has got greenfly on it. You have to get rid of the greenfly.' The Jews weren't human beings for them. It was like killing fleas." Hitler had well prepared for the mentality: Jews were portrayed by him as "parasites, cankers, worthless, germ carriers, a lower species." Lifton, *The Nazi Doctors*, 16.

34. The Washington State Medical Association, with other organizations, has published a 236-page manual, *Pain Management and the Care of the Terminal Patient*, which can be obtained from the association at 2033 Sixth Avenue, Suite 900, Seattle, Washington 98121. Much has been written on the distinction between "passive euthanasia" (allowing to die) and "active euthanasia" (intentionally killing). Some of the various positions appear in B. Steinbock, ed., *Killing and Letting Die* (Englewood Cliffs, N.J.: Prentice-Hall, 1980)—especially the articles by Rachels and Davis. Rachels has written his own work, *The End of Life: Euthanasia and Morality* (New York: Oxford University Press, 1987). Derek Humphry, with A. Wickett, makes his own defense in *The Right To Die: Understanding Euthanasia* (New York: Harper and Row, 1986).

   The "double effect" argument—that one cannot directly intend an evil but might place a good or neutral act that brings about an unintended evil, as long as the "evil" is not the cause of the desired good (i.e., "The end does not justify the means")—was unsuccessfully challenged by Miner in the Second Circuit U.S. Court of Appeals judgment in *Quill v. Vacco*, 80 F.3d 716 (1996). Miner claimed that assisted suicide was the same as withdrawal or withholding of treatment. Ironically, Miner noted that conservative Supreme Court Justice Scalia agreed—despite the overwhelming evidence that because withdrawal of treatment often does not lead to death, it cannot possibly be *equated with* the intent to kill.

NOTES TO CHAPTER EIGHT

1. Robert Nozick, *The Examined Life: Philosophical Meditations* (New York: Simon and Schuster, 1989), 131–32. Nozick's political philosophy, which is developed in *Anarchy, State and Utopia* (Oxford: Basil Blackwell, 1974), is a strong natural rights theory, nonutilitarian, which gives a high value to property rights in a manner that is not entirely congenial to the radical personalism offered here. A personalist political and economic ethic would be grounded on the conviction of the primacy of persons over property, the primacy of labor over capital.

2. Fyodor Dostoyevsky, *The Brothers Karamazov* (New York: Modern Library, 1996), Chapter 4, "A Lady of Little Faith."

3. Donald Katz, "Men, Women & Money: the Last Taboo," *Worth*, June 1993, 55–56.

4. Rainer Maria Rilke, *Letters to a Young Poet*, trans. M. D. Herter Norton (New York: Norton, 1963), 69.

5. Ian Mitroff and Warren Bennis, *The Unreality Industry* (New York: Birch Lane Press, 1989)—aptly subtitled "The Deliberate Manufacturing of Falsehood and What It Is Doing to Our Lives"—asks the question: "What can the fate

of any society be that has to function in a complex world if its fundamental reason for being has degenerated into the production and consumption of limitless amounts of unreality?" (20). A fascinating critique of the "constructed" cultural reality of media and entertainment, it could be strengthened by a greater probing of the role of capitalism in this unreal world. For a wholly different but ironically confirming approach, see Camille Paglia's wacky *Sex, Art, and American Culture* (New York: Vintage, 1992). Because Paglia seems deadly serious about her interpretations, her work and her public persona represent a chilling theoretical rationalization of cultural pretense.

6. Katz, "Men, Women & Money." I am amazed that so many academics—of the left and the right—who stress "heritage," "culture,'" and "social construction" as powerfully formative on the notion of self and codes of life seem utterly innocent of the influence of capitalism on their own ethical pronouncements, their philosophies, or their approach to life. David Rieff, in "Multiculturalism's Silent Partner: It's the New Globalized Consumer Economy, Stupid," *Harper's*, August 1993, is one of the few to point out how the great "diversification" in academic life is so amenable to capitalism:

> Once administrators have decided that the university will be a kind of department store, then each new course offering becomes little more than another product line, and department chairpersons begin to act like the store's buyers. . . .
>
> Perhaps it's tenure, with its way of shielding the senior staff from the rigors of someone else's bottom line thinking. Working for an institution in which neither pay nor promotion is connected to performance, job security is guaranteed (after tenure is attained), and pension arrangements are probably the finest in any industry in the country—no wonder a poststructuralist can easily believe that words are deeds (63, 66).

A refreshing exception to academia's seemingly uncritical acceptance of market forces at work in the profession is Patrick Murray's *Reflections on Commercial Life: An Anthology of Classic Texts from Plato to the Present* (New York: Routledge, 1997). Although the entire collection is outstanding, the general introduction is unequaled in its analysis of the ways that capitalism has embedded itself in the symbolic and practical "forms" of our lives.

7. Robert Louden offers a theoretical counterpart to this position in *Morality and Moral Theory* (New York: Oxford, 1992). Louden emphasizes the moral agent: the kind of person one is. Although he does not present a full-blown ethical position, it clearly would have strong Kantian and Aristotelian themes, with emphasis on the "virtue" approach to ethics (see note 17). A more popularized counterpart appears in Alfie Kohn, *The Brighter Side of Human Nature: Altruism and Empathy in Everyday Life* (New York: Basic Books, 1990).

8. James Twitchell, *Lead Us Into Temptation* (New York: Columbia University Press, 1999). The extended quotation is from pages 284–86. Earlier references are to pages 12, 30–31, and 49.

   Two somewhat popularized accounts of the relationship between cultural "reality" and personal identity are Walter Truett Anderson's *Reality Isn't What It Used To Be* (San Francisco: Harper, 1990) and Kenneth Gergen's *The Saturated Self: Dilemmas of Identity in Contemporary Life* (New York: Basic Books, 1991). Richard Stivers' *The Culture of Cynicism* (Cambridge: Blackwell, 1994) is a stimulating analysis from the viewpoint of moral and social theory. Jacob Needleman, one of the few philosophers to investigate the power of money-capitalism in the formation of our ethos and spirits, writes, "Weren't most of us sternly admonished at a very tender age to save our money, to be so very careful with it—to such an extent that we grew up feeling, if not consciously thinking that our relationship to money was the source of our value and worthiness as a human being? For many of us, money was the most real thing is life, and therefore the most sacred thing." *Money and the Meaning of Life* (New York: Doubleday, 1991), 267.

9. "Behind the Fly: Bono—The Interview," *Rolling Stone*, March 4, 1993, 42–45.

10. Russell Belk, Melanie Wallendorf, and John Sherry, "The Sacred and the Profane in Consumer Behavior: Theodicy on the Odyssey," *Journal of Consumer Research* 16 (June 1989): 2. See also William Kowinski, *The Malling of America: An Insider Look at the Great Consumer Paradise* (New York: W. Morrow, 1985). A more recent—and telling—article is David Guterson's "Enclosed, Encyclopedic, Endured: One Week at the Mall of America," *Harper's*, August 1993, 49–56: "The mall was five times larger than Red Square and twenty times larger than St. Peter's Basilica. . . ."

11. The strange quality of our relationship to possessions is treated with historical scope in James Lincoln Collier, *The Rise of Selfishness in America* (New York: Oxford, 1991). Collier's work is an invaluable resource in understanding America's social history, especially in the context of material prosperity, the media and entertainment, and their relationship with personal identity and social cohesion. On a global scale, Alan Durning's *How Much Is Enough? The Consumer Society and the Future of the Earth* (New York: Norton, 1992) investigates the international and ecological implications of "capitalist" reality: "In the final analysis, accepting and living by sufficiency rather than excess offers a return to what is, culturally speaking, the human home: to the ancient order of family, community, good work, and a good life; to a reverence for skill, creativity, and creation; to a daily cadence slow enough to let us watch the sunset and stroll by the water's edge; to communities worth spending a lifetime in; and to local places pregnant with memories of generations" (150).

Appropriately, as the 1980s began, Philip Slater offered the slim volume *Wealth Addiction* (New York: Dutton, 1980). The section on "reconnecting" begins with "All addictions are more or less alike. It doesn't really matter what you're addicted to; they all involve some feeling of deficiency: 'I will be complete only if I have X.' I have defined addiction as a perceived hole in the self which can be filled only by taking something in from the world. Obviously, then, all cures are also alike. They all involve finding some way to say 'I am complete *without* X'" (164). Halfway through the decade, Laurence Shames saw not much of a cure in *The Hunger for More: Searching for Values in an Age of Greed* (New York: Vintage, 1986): "The confusion of realms, finally, was what made the apotheosis of the marketplace a grim prospect. The encroachment by the marketplace definition of worth on the broader notion of worthiness; the annexation of the whole realm of values by the marketplace version of value—those were reductions that made life poorer" (194).

Harvard's Juliet Schor has offered two strong critiques of consumerism: *The Overworked American* (New York: Basic Books, 1992) and *The Overspent American* (New York: Basic Books, 1998).

12. Karl Marx, *Capital, I,* trans. Samuel Moore and Edward Aveling (New York: International Publishers, 1967), 72. Sut Jhally develops the theme of fetishism in *The Codes of Advertising: Fetishism and the Political Economy of Meaning in the Consumer Society* (New York: Routledge, 1990). The "fetish" relation continues after the product is taken home. The clothes tag for Vanity Fair lingerie reads, "The philosophy? That lingerie should touch more than a woman's body when she slips it on. . . . it should touch her soul." The tag for Laura Ashley promises an even more intense relationship: "Our purpose is to establish an enduring relationship with those who share a love of the special lifestyle that is Laura Ashley. We will act to protect the integrity of that relationship and to ensure its long-term prosperity."

Some of the material in this section is based on an audiovisual presentation "Advertising and the Formation of Consciousness" that I gave in lectures over several years. They appear, in slightly shorter and altered form, in the Canadian "alternative media" journal *Adbusters* 2, no. 3 (winter 1993): 18–22. The entire issue (which was published by The Media Foundation, 1243 West 7th Ave., Vancouver, British Columbia) was about religion and advertising. I offered the same article—under the title "New Time Religion: Accept Consumerism in Your Heart"—to some business ethics classes and faculty seminars at Saint John's University in spring 1993 as part of the visiting McKeever Chair in Moral Theology.

13. The parallels between contemporary extravaganzas in "superdomes" and the rallies of the Third Reich have also been noted in Douglas Rushkoff's fascinating *Coercion: Why We Listen To What "They" Say* (New York: Penguin Putnam, 1999), especially chapters three and five.

14. Needleman, *Money and the Meaning of Life*, 165. "The determining characteristic of our modern era has been the unprecedented extent to which the inner ideals embodied in traditional patterns of human relationship—for example, family duty, care for the well-being and dignity of one's neighbor, and respect for life, with all the subtle refinements of behavior and perception that have been associated with these values over the centuries—no longer seem inwardly intense and vivid" (157).

   In mainline academic ethics, Elizabeth Anscombe's essay "Modern Moral Philosophy," *Philosophy* 33 (1958): 1–19, raised the possibility that ethical theory was ineffectual because it had neglected the character issue of the "kind" of human one ought to be. This argument led to a renewed interest in "virtue" theory and in philosophical anthropology. To discover what kind of life and practices a fully functioning person might exhibit, the question of human nature was raised once again. More recently, MacIntyre's *After Virtue* related the issue of virtue to the cultural heritage in which men and women find themselves. Complaining that modern consciousness offers no coherent moral heritage, MacIntyre commends the Aristotelian and Thomistic "traditions," not for their metaphysics or philosophical anthropologies but for their approaches to "good" and "virtue." As I have suggested in earlier chapters of this book, I suspect that any discussion of virtue or good must be grounded in a philosophy of personal human nature.

15. *Walden and Civil Disobedience* (New York: Penguin, 1983 [1854]), 135. Thoreau's comments on academic professionals are worth noting: "There are nowadays professors of philosophy, but not philosophers. Yet it is admirable to profess because it was once admirable to live. To be a philosopher is not merely to have subtle thoughts, nor even to found a school, but so to love wisdom as to live according to its dictates, a life of simplicity, independence, magnanimity and trust. It is to solve some of the problems of life, not only theoretically, but practically" (57).

16. The fruitfulness of solitude has struck a chord in contemporary consciousness, as the response to Thomas Moore's *Care of the Soul: A Guide for Cultivating Depth and Sacredness in Everyday Life* (New York: Harper Collins, 1992) attests. On the theoretical level, the growing interest in the philosophy of "spirituality" is indicated by the publication of Joel Kovel's *History and Spirit: An Inquiry into the Philosophy of Liberation* (Boston: Beacon Press, 1991)—a sympathetic inquiry into the meaning of "spirit" from the viewpoint of a nonbeliever.

17. Leo Tolstoy, *The Death of Ivan Ilyitch and Other Stories*, trans. Aylmer Maude (New York: New American Library, 1960), 132–33.

18. William F. May, *The Patient's Ordeal* (Bloomington: Indiana University Press, 1994), 205. This brilliant and courageous treatment of human suffer-

ing closes with an appeal that all professionals, including clergy, face honestly the horrific pain that profoundly damaged persons experience.

19. Daniel Callahan, *The Troubled Dream of Life: In Search of a Peaceful Death* (Washington, D.C.: Georgetown University Press, 2000). This book may be the most significant work of a much-published and pioneering medical ethicist. Callahan affirms the dignity of the human person, even in dying, and effectively challenges the belief that all treatments must be undertaken or sustained.

20. Dostoyevsky, *The Brothers Karamazov*.

21. Dorothy Day writes of self-critique frequently in her autobiographical journals; it is powerfully evident in Robert Coles' brilliant study, *Dorothy Day: A Radical Devotion* (Reading, Mass.: Addison-Wesley, 1987). Mother Teresa's remark was made in a personal conversation. Jean Vanier—the man who, soon after receiving his doctoral degree, started the L'Arche communities for the handicapped—writes of self-critique in *Community and Growth: Our Pilgrimage Together* (New York: Paulist Press, 1979). Simone Weil, a brilliant philosopher, also addressed this notion; see Eric Springsted's edition of *Simone Weil* (Maryknoll, N.Y.: Orbis, 1988).

   Samuel and Pearl Oliner, *The Altruistic Personality: Rescuers of Jews in Nazi Europe* (New York: Macmillan, 1988), note that the "habit" of committed personal intimacy clearly was central in the heroic response to moral crisis: "Rescuers, like nonrescuers, worried both before and during the war about feeding, sheltering, and protecting themselves and their families. What distinguished rescuers was not their lack of concern with self, external approval, or achievement, but rather their capacity for extensive relationships—their stronger sense of attachment to others and their feeling of responsibility for the welfare of others, including those outside their immediate familial or communal circles. . . . It begins in close family relationships in which parents model caring behavior and communicate caring values" (248).

22. "Choosing Death," *The Health Quarterly*, March 23, 1995. Herbert Hendin, M.D., probes the paradoxes of "care" and lack of it in the Dutch euthanaesia experience in *Seduced by Death* (New York: Norton, 1997). Two powerfully moving presentations of the contrasts between personal engagement and professional depersonalization in health care are Frank Huyler's *The Blood of Strangers: Stories from Emergency Medicine* (Berkeley: University of California Press, 1999) and Margaret Edson's Pulitzer Prize-winning *Wit: A Play* (New York: Farrar, Straus & Giroux, 1999).

23. Buber's *I and Thou* (London: Routledge, 1942) and *Between Man and Man* (London: Routledge, 1947) and *The Letters of Martin Buber: A Life of Dialogue*, ed. Nahum Glatzer and Paul Mendes-Flohr (New York: Schocken, 1991) are preeminent contemporary examples. In the philosophy of "otherness," the

works of Max Scheler, Emmanuel Levinas, Enrique Dussell in "liberation philosophy," and Alfred Schutz and Maurice Natanson in phenomenology have had considerable influence. Moreover, just as there are "meditative," "confessional," and autobiographical traditions in philosophy, there also is a "dialogical" tradition—from Plato through the disputation style of Thomas Aquinas to Hume's dialogues concerning religion.

24. Oliver Sacks has such great power as a clinician and writer because he enters so empathetically into the personal reality of his most damaged patients. His respect and love for them—"the noblest people I have ever known"—is matched only by the philosophical and neurological scope of his knowledge. This is especially evident in his brilliant *Awakenings* (New York: Harper Perennial, 1990).

25. Coles frequented the "Catholic Worker" house for the homeless while he was studying medicine, and his academic work has the unmistakable "feel" of someone who has entered the reality of the marginal people he has worked with. See, for example, *Migrants, Sharecroppers, Mountaineers* (Boston: Little, Brown, 1971) and *Children of Crisis: A Study of Courage and Fear* (Boston: Little, Brown, 1967). In this context of marginality and the professorate, I particularly recommend Patricia Williams, "Owning the Self in a Disowned World," in *The Alchemy of Race and Rights* (Cambridge, Mass.: Harvard University Press, 1991). When Williams was associate professor of law at the University of Wisconsin, she wrote of the anguish in integrating disparate realities—the academic profession, the media world, being black and woman, theory and life: "After a while I turn off the television and pick up the newspaper. I think to find solace there, but the world gets weirder and weirder all the time" (186).

26. See *Night* by Elie Wiesel, foreword by Francois Mauriac (New York: Avon Books, 1969), and Viktor Frankl's *Man's Search For Meaning* (Boston: Beacon Press, 1962) and *The Doctor and the Soul* (New York: Knopf, 1965). A treatment of the dangers inherent in "pure theory" separated from human suffering appears in Christopher Norris' *Uncritical Theory: Postmodernism, Intellectuals, and The Gulf War* (Amherst: University of Massachusetts Press, 1992).

27. Jean-Dominique Bauby, *The Diving Bell and the Butterfly*, trans. Jeremy Leggatt (New York: Alfred A. Knopf, 1997), 70, 71.

28. This passage appears in a catalogue of her photographs, *Mev Puleo: Witness to Life* (St. Louis: Samuel Cupples House and McNamee Gallery, 1997), 11. Shortly before her death, Puleo also authored *The Struggle is One: Voices and Visions of Liberation* (Albany: SUNY Press, 1994).

29. Sheila Cassidy, "Hospices: A Prophetic Moment," in *Spiritual Journeys*, ed. Stanislaus Kennedy (Dublin: Veritas, 1997), 163.

30. A major theme of Ernest Becker's work is the fear and denial of our creatureliness not only as the source of our lack of self-knowledge but also

as the drive behind violence. "All power is in essence power to deny mortality. . . . Power means to increase oneself, to change one's natural situation from one of smallness, helplessness, finitude, to one of bigness, control, durability, importance." *Escape from Evil* (New York: Free Press, 1975), 81.

31. Danielle Darriet, *Bulletin* (Institute for Theological Enclounter with Science and Technology) 28, no. 2 (spring 1997) (lecture originally given at Catholic Student Center of Washington University, St. Louis).

32. Jean Vanier, "Understanding our own Brokenness," in *Spiritual Journeys*, 15.

33. Taylor, *Sources of the Self*, 518.

34. John Macmurray did not consider such a statement "idealism." He called it "sober realism," even though it was uttered during the onset of World War II during the Foundation Address at University College, London. I am grateful to Jack Costello, president of Regis College in Toronto and Macmurray scholar, for informing me about this Macmurray lecture.

Bibliography

African Rights. *Rwanda: Death, Despair and Defiance*. London: African Rights, 1995.

Allen, Woody, director. *Crimes and Misdemeanors*. Orion Films, 1989.

Anderson, Walter Truett. *Reality Isn't What it Used to Be*. San Francisco: Harper & Row, 1990.

Anscombe, Elizabeth. "Modern Moral Philosophy." *Philosophy* 33 (1958): 1–19.

Ayer, A.J. *Language, Truth and Logic*. London: Gollancz, 1936.

Baars, Bernard J. *In the Theater of Consciousness*. New York: Oxford University Press, 1997.

Baillie, James. *Problems in Personal Identity*. New York: Paragon House, 1993.

Barrett, William. *The Death of the Soul*. New York: Doubleday, 1986.

Barrow, Robin. *Utilitarianism: A Contemporary Statement*. Brookfield, Vt.: Edward Elgar, 1991.

Bauby, Jean-Dominique. *The Diving Bell and the Butterfly*. Translated by Jeremy Leggatt. New York: Alfred A. Knopf, 1997.

Baynes, Kenneth, James Bohman, and Thomas McCarthy, eds. *After Philosophy: End or Transformation?* Cambridge, Mass.: MIT Press, 1988.

Beauchamp, Tom L., and James F. Childress, eds. *Principles of Biomedical Ethics*. 3rd edition. New York: Oxford University Press, 1989.

Beck, Lewis White. *A Commentary on Kant's Critique of Pure Reason*. Chicago: University of Chicago Press, 1960.

Becker, Ernest. *Escape from Evil*. New York: Free Press, 1975.

Bedau, Hugo Adam. *Studies in the Morality, Law, and Politics of Capital Punishment*. Boston: Northeastern University Press, 1987.

Bellah, Robert, et al. *The Good Society*. New York: Alfred A. Knopf, 1991.

———. *Habits of the Heart*. New York: Harper & Row, 1985.

Benhabib, Seyla. *Situating the Self*. New York: Routledge, 1992.

Bernstein, Richard J. *Beyond Objectivism and Relativism: Science, Hermeneutics, and Praxis*. Philadelphia: University of Pennsylvania Press, 1983.

———. *The New Constellation: The Ethical-Political Horizons of Modernity/Postmodernity*. Cambridge, Mass.: MIT Press, 1991.

———. *Philosophical Profiles*. New York: Cambridge University Press, 1986.

Berry, Christopher. *Human Nature*. Atlantic City, N.J.: Humanities Press, 1986.

Bourke, Vernon J. *Ethics*, 2nd ed. New York: Macmillan Co., 1966.

Brink, David. *Moral Realism and the Foundation of Ethics*. New York: Cambridge University Press, 1989.

Brody, Baruch. *Abortion and the Sanctity of Human Life: A Philosophical View*. Cambridge, Mass.: MIT Press, 1975.

Bruner, Jerome. *Acts of Meaning*. Cambridge, Mass.: Harvard University Press, 1990.

Buber, Martin. *I and Thou*. London: Routledge, 1947.

———. *Between Man and Man*. London: Routledge, 1947.

———. *The Letters of Martin Buber: A Life of Dialogue*. Edited by Nahum Glatzer and Paul Mendes-Flohr. New York: Schocken, 1991.

Cahoone, Lawrence E. *The Dilemma of Modernity*. Albany, N.Y.: SUNY Press, 1988.

Callahan, Daniel. *The Troubled Dream Life: In Search of a Peaceful Death*. Washington, D.C.: Georgetown University Press, 2000.

Camus, Albert. *The Fall*. Translated by Justin O'Brien. New York: Vintage Books, 1956.

———. *The Myth of Sisyphus & Other Stories*. New York: Vintage, 1991.

———. *The Plague*. New York: Vintage, 1991.

———. *The Rebel*. New York: Vintage, 1991.

———. *The Stranger*. New York: Vintage, 1989.

Carney, James Guadalupe. *To Be a Revolutionary*. New York: Harper & Row, 1987.

Carruthers, Peter. *Introducing Persons*. Albany, N.Y.: SUNY Press, 1986.

Cassidy, Sheila. "Hospices: A Prophetic Moment." In *Spiritual Journeys*. Edited by Stanislaus Kennedy. Dublin: Veritas, 1997.

Cheney, Dorothy, and Robert Seyfarth. *How Monkeys See the World: Inside the Mind of Another Species*. Chicago: University of Chicago Press, 1990.

Christensen, Scott, and Dale Turner, eds. *Folk Psychology and the Philosophy of Mind*. Hillsdale, N.J.: Erlbaum, 1993.

Christman, John, ed. *Autonomy, the Inner Citadel*. New York: Oxford University Press, 1989.

Churchland, Patricia. *Neurophilosophy: Toward a Unified Science of the Mind-Brain*. Cambridge, Mass.: MIT Press, 1986.

Clark, Eric. *The Want Makers*. New York: Viking, 1989.

Coles, Robert. *Children of Crisis: A Study of Courage and Fear*. Boston: Little, Brown, 1967.

———. *Migrants, Sharecroppers, Mountaineers*. Boston: Little, Brown, 1971.

Collier, James Lincoln. *The Rise of Selfishness in America*. New York: Oxford University Press, 1991.

Collins, James. *A History of Modern European Philosophy*. Milwaukee, Wisc.: Bruce Publishing, 1954.

Copleston, Frederick. *A History of Philosophy*. Three volumes. Garden City, N.Y.: Image Books, 1985.

Crossette, Barbara. "Civilians Will be in Harm's Way if Baghdad is Hit." *New York Times*, January 28, 1998.

Daly, Mary. *Gyn/Ecology: The Metaethics of Radical Feminism*. Boston: Beacon Press, 1978.

Damasio, Antonio. *Descartes' Error: Emotion, Reason and the Human Brain*. New York: Putnam, 1994.

———. *The Feeling of What Happens*. New York: Harcourt, Brace & Company, 1999.

Darriet, Danielle. *Bulletin* (Institute for Theological Encounter with Science and Technology) 28 (1997).

Day, Dorothy. *Dorothy Day: A Radical Devotion*. Reading, Mass.: Addison-Wesley, 1987.

Dennett, Daniel. *Brainstorms: Philosophical Essays on Mind and Psychology*. Cambridge, Mass.: MIT Press, 1986.

———. *Consciousness Explained*. New York: Little, Brown, 1992.

Dillard, Annie. *For the Time Being*. New York: Alfred A. Knopf, 1999.

Dombrowski, Daniel. *Babies and Beasts: The Argument from Marginal Cases*. Chicago: University of Illinois Press, 1997.

Donagan, Alan. *The Theory of Morality*. Chicago: University of Chicago Press, 1977.

Doran, Kevin. *What Is a Person? The Concept and Implications for Ethics*. Lewiston, N.Y.: Edwin Mellon Press, 1989.

Dostoievsky, Fyodor. *The Brothers Karamazov*. New York: Modern Library, 1996.

D'Souza, Dinesh. *Illiberal Education*. New York: Free Press, 1991.

Durning, Alan. *How Much is Enough? The Consumer Society and the Future of the Earth*. New York: W. W. Norton, 1992.

Dworkin, Ronald. *Life's Dominion: An Argument about Abortion, Euthanasia, and Individual Freedom*. New York: Alfred A. Knopf, 1993.

Edelman, Gerald. *Bright Air, Brilliant Fire: On the Matter of the Mind*. New York: Basic Books, 1992.

Edsen, Margaret. *Wit: A Play*. New York: Farrar Straus & Giroux, 1999.

Ewen, Stuart. *All Consuming Images*. New York: Basic Books, 1988.

Finnis, John. *Fundamentals of Ethics*. Washington, D.C.: Georgetown University Press, 1983.

———. *Natural Law and Natural Rights*. Oxford: Clarendon Press, 1982.

Fischer, Louis, ed. *The Essential Gandhi*. New York: Vintage, 1963.

Flanagan, Owen. *Consciousness Reconsidered*. Cambridge, Mass.: MIT Press, 1992.

Ford, Norman. *When Did I Begin? Conception of the Human Individual in History, Philosophy and Science*. New York: Cambridge University Press, 1991.

Frank, Robert. *Luxury Fever*. New York: Free Press, 1999.

Frankl, Viktor. *The Doctor and the Soul*. New York: Alfred A. Knopf, 1965.

————. *Man's Search for Meaning*. Boston: Beacon Press, 1962.

Fraser, Nancy. "Solidarity or Singularity? Richard Rorty Between Romanticism and Technocracy." *Praxis International* 8 (1988).

French, Marilyn. *The War Against Women*. New York: Ballantine, 1992.

Freud, Sigmund. *Civilization and Its Discontents*. Translated and edited by James Strachey. New York: W. W. Norton, 1961.

————. *The Future of an Illusion*. New York: W. W. Norton, 1961.

————. *New Introductory Lectures on Psycho-Analysis*. Translated by W. J. H. Sprott. New York: W. W. Norton, 1933.

Gallie, W. B., ed. *Philosophers of Peace and War: Kant, Clausewitz, Marx, Engels and Tolstoy*. New York: Cambridge University Press, 1978.

Gasche, Rodolphe, *The Tain of the Mirror*. Cambridge, Mass.: Harvard University Press, 1986.

Gates, Henry Louis, Jr. "A Liberalism of Heart and Spine." *New York Times*, March 27, 1994.

Gergen, Kenneth. *The Saturated Self: Dilemmas of Identity in Contemporary Life*. New York: Basic Books, 1991.

Giddens, Anthony. *Modernity and Self-Identity: Self and Society in the Late Modern Age*. Stanford, Calif.: Stanford University Press, 1991.

Gilligan, Carol. *In a Different Voice: Psychological Theory and Women's Development*. Cambridge, Mass.: Harvard University Press, 1982.

Goodall, Jane. *Through a Window: My Thirty Years with the Chimpanzees of Gombe*. Boston: Houghton Mifflin, 1990.

Grisez, Germain, and Russell Shaw. *Beyond the New Morality*. Notre Dame, Ind.: University of Notre Dame Press, 1980.

Grossman, Dave. *On Killing: The Psychological Cost of Learning to Kill in War and Society*. Boston: Little, Brown, 1995.

Guterson, David. "Enclosed, Encyclopedic, Endured: One Week at the Mall of America." *Harper's*, August 1993, 49–56.

Guyer, Paul, ed. *The Cambridge Companion to Kant*. New York: Cambridge University Press, 1992.

Haber, Joram Graf, ed. *Absolutism and its Consequentialist Critics*. Lanham, Md.: Rowman and Littlefield, 1994.

Hallett, Garth. *Christian Moral Reasoning: An Analytic Guide*. Notre Dame, Ind.: University of Notre Dame Press, 1983.

————. *Reason and Right*. Notre Dame, Ind.: University of Notre Dame Press, 1984.

Hanink, James, "The Personalist Vision." *New Oxford Review* (1989): 6–11.

Harre, Ron. *Personal Being*. Cambridge, Mass.: Harvard University Press, 1984.

Havel, Vaclav. "The End of the Modern Era." *New York Times*, March 1, 1992.

Hendin, Herbert, M.D. *Seduced by Death*. New York: W. W. Norton, 1997.

Hopkins, Gerard Manley. *The Poems of Gerard Manley Hopkins.* Edited by W. H. Gardner and N. H. MacKenzie. New York: Oxford University Press, 1970.

Horgan, John. *The Undiscovered Mind.* New York: Free Press, 1999.

Hughes, Robert. *The Culture of Complaint: The Fraying of America.* New York: Oxford University Press, 1993.

Human Rights Watch. *Slaughter Among Neighbors.* New Haven, Conn.: Yale University Press, 1995.

Hume, David. *A Treatise of Human Nature.* Edited by L. A. Selby-Bigge and P. H. Nidditch. Oxford: Clarendon Press, 1978.

Humphry, Derek. *Final Exit.* Eugene, Ore.: Hemlock Society, 1991.

Humphry, Derek, and A. Wickett. *The Right to Die: Understanding Euthanasia.* New York: Harper and Row, 1986.

Huyler, Frank. *The Blood of Strangers: Stories from Emergency Medicine.* Berkeley: University of California Press, 1999.

Jaggar, Allison. *Feminist Politics and Human Nature.* Totowa, N.J.: Rowman & Littlefield, 1983.

Jhally, Sut. *The Codes of Advertising: Fetishism and the Political Economy of Meaning in the Consumer Society.* New York: Routledge, 1990.

Johnson, James Turner, and John Kelsay, eds. *Cross, Crescent and Sword: The Justification and Limitation of War in Western and Islamic Traditions.* New York: Greenwood Press, 1990.

Kaelin, E. F., and C. O. Schrag, eds. *Analecta Husserliana*, Vol. XXVI. Boston: Kluwer Academic Publishers, 1989.

Kainz, Howard P. *Philosophical Perspectives on Peace: An Anthology of Classical and Modern Sources.* Athens, Ohio: Ohio University Press, 1987.

Kant, Immanuel. *Fundamental Principles of the Metaphysics of Morals.* Translated by T. K. Abbott. In *Kant's Theory of Ethics*, 4th ed. London: Longmans, Green & Co., 1990.

Katz, Donald. "Men, Women & Money: The Last Taboo." *Worth*, June 1993, 55–56.

Kavanaugh, John, S.J. "Advertising and the Formation of Consciousness." *Adbusters* 2 (1993): 18–22.

———. "What Is It Like to Be Bats or Brains? Similarities and Differences between Humans and Other Animals." *Modern Schoolman* 76 (1998).

———. "Intrinsic Values, Persons and Stewardship." In *The Challenge of Global Stewardship: Roman Catholic Responses.* Edited by Maura Ryan and Todd Whitmore. Notre Dame, Ind.: University of Notre Dame Press, 1997.

Keen, Sam. *Faces of the Enemy: Reflections of the Hostile Imagination.* San Francisco: Harper & Row, 1986.

Keller, Helen. *The Story of My Life.* New York: Airmont Books, 1965.

Kenny, Anthony. *The Metaphysics of Mind.* Oxford: Clarendon Press, 1989.

Kevorkian, Jack. *Prescription Medicine: The Goodness of Planned Death.* Buffalo, N.Y.: Prometheus Books, 1991.

Kierkegaard, Soren. *The Sickness Unto Death.* Translated by Walter Lowrie. Princeton, N.J.: Princeton University Press, 1951.

Kimbrell, Andrew. *The Human Body Shop: The Engineering and Marketing of Life.* San Francisco: Harper & Row, 1993.

King, Rev. Dr. Martin Luther, Jr. "Letter from a Birmingham Jail." In *Why We Can't Wait.* New York: Harper, 1963.

Kleinig, John. *Valuing Life.* Princeton, N.J.: Princeton University Press, 1991.

Klubertanz, George. *Habits and Virtues.* New York: Appleton-Century-Crofts, 1965.

———. *Philosophy of Human Nature.* New York: Appleton-Century-Crofts, 1953.

Kohlberg, Lawrence. *The Philosophy of Moral Development: Moral Stages and the Idea of Justice.* San Francisco: Harper & Row, 1981.

Kohn, Alfie. *The Brighter Side of Human Nature: Altruism and Empathy in Everyday Life.* New York: Basic Books, 1990.

Kovel, Joel. *History and Spirit: An Inquiry into the Philosophy of Liberation.* Boston: Beacon Press, 1991.

Kowinski, William. *The Malling of America: An Insider Look at the Great Consumer Paradise.* New York: William Morrow, 1985.

Kretzmann, Norman, and Eleonore Stump, eds. *The Cambridge Companion to Aquinas.* New York: Cambridge University Press, 1993.

Lasch, Christopher. *The Culture of Narcissism.* New York: W. W. Norton, 1979.

———. *The Minimal Self.* New York: W. W. Norton, 1984.

———. *The True and Only Heaven.* New York: W. W. Norton, 1991.

Leland, Doris. "Rorty on the Moral Concern of Philosophy: A Critique from a Feminist Point of View." *Praxis International* 8 (1988).

Lewis, C. S. *The Abolition of Man.* New York: Macmillan, 1947.

———. *Studies in Words.* New York: Cambridge University Press, 1960.

Lifton, Robert Jay. *The Nazi Doctors.* New York: Basic Books, 1986.

Lisska, Anthony. *Aquinas' Theory of Law: An Analytic Reconstruction.* Oxford: Clarendon, 1996.

Loewy, Erich H. "Harming, Healing, and Euthanasia." In *Regulating How We Die.* Edited by Linda Emanuel. Cambridge, Mass.: Harvard University Press, 1998.

Lonergan, Bernard. *Insight: A Study of Human Understanding.* New York: Philosophical Library, 1958.

Louden, Robert. *Morality and Moral Theory.* New York: Oxford, 1992.

Luijpen, William. *Phenomenology of Natural Law.* Pittsburgh: Duquesne University Press, 1967.

MacDonald, Scott, and Eleonore Stump, eds. *Aquinas' Moral Theory.* Ithaca, N.Y.: Cornell University Press, 1999.

MacIntyre, Alasdair. *After Virtue*. Notre Dame, Ind.: University of Notre Dame Press, 1984.

———. *Dependent Rational Animals: Why Human Beings Need the Virtues*. Chicago: Open Court, 1999.

———. *Whose Justice? Which Rationality?* Notre Dame, Ind.: University of Notre Dame Press, 1989.

Mackie, J. L. *Ethics: Inventing Right and Wrong*. Harmondsworth, England: Penguin, 1977.

Macmurray, John. "Foundation Address." *The New Community* (April 1941), 68–80.

———. *Freedom in the Modern World*. New York: Harper & Row, 1961.

———. *Persons in Relation*. London: Faber & Faber, 1935.

———. *The Self as Agent*. New York: Humanities Press, 1978 [1957].

Manent, Pierre. *The City of Man*. Princeton, N.J.: Princeton University Press, 1998.

Manning, Rita C. *Speaking from the Heart: A Feminist Perspective on Ethics*. Lanham, Md.: Rowman & Littlefield, 1992.

Marcuse, Herbert. *Five Lectures*. Translated by J. Shapiro and S. Weber. Boston: Beacon Press, 1968.

Marsh, James. *Post-Cartesian Meditations*. New York: Fordham University Press, 1988.

Marx, Karl. *Capital I*. Translated by Moore and Aveling. New York: International Publishers, 1967.

Maslow, Abraham. *Toward a Psychology of Being*. 2nd ed. Princeton, N.J.: Van Nostrand Insight Books, 1962.

May, Gerald G., M.D. *Will and Spirit: A Contemplative Psychology*. San Francisco: Harper & Row, 1982.

May, Rollo. *Love and Will*. New York: Delta, 1964.

———. *Freud and Man's Soul*. New York: Vintage, 1984.

———. *Psychology and the Human Dilemma*. New York: Van Nostrand, 1967.

May, William F. *The Patient's Ordeal*. Bloomington: Indiana University Press, 1994.

McCarthy, Michael. *The Crisis of Philosophy*. Albany: State University of New York Press, 1990.

McCarthy, Thomas. "Private Irony and Public Decency: Richard Rorty's New Pragmatism." *Critical Inquiry* 16 (1990): 355–70.

McChesney, Robert. *Rich Media, Poor Democracy*. Urbana: University of Illinois Press, 1999.

McCulloch, Gregory. *The Mind and Its World*. London: Routledge, 1995.

McGinn, Colin, ed. *Minds and Bodies: Philosophers and Their Ideas*. New York: Oxford University Press, 1997.

———. *The Mysterious Flame*. New York: Basic Books, 1999.

McInerny, Ralph. *Aquinas on Human Action: A Theory of Practice*. Washington, D.C.: Catholic University of America Press, 1992.

McVeigh, Timothy. "An Essay on Hypocrisy." *Media Bypass Magazine*, June 1998.

Merleau-Ponty, Maurice. *The Essential Writings of Merleau-Ponty*. Edited by Alden L. Fisher. New York: Harcourt, Brace & World, 1969.

————. *The Structure of Behavior*. Boston: Beacon Press, 1963.

Midgley, Mary. *Can't We Make Moral Judgements?* New York: Saint Martin's Press, 1991.

Mill, John Stuart. *On Liberty*, in *Collected Works*, Volume 10. Toronto: University of Toronto Press, 1969.

————. *Utilitarianism*, in *Collected Works*, Volume 10. Toronto: University of Toronto Press, 1969.

Miller, Mark Crispin. *Boxed In: The Culture of TV*. Evanston, Ill.: Northwestern University Press, 1988.

Minsky, Marvin. *Society of Mind*. New York: Simon and Schuster, 1985.

Mitroff, Ian, and Warren Bennis. *The Unreality Industry*. New York: Birch Lane Press, 1989.

Moore, Thomas. *Care of the Soul: A Guide for Cultivating Depth and Sacredness in Everyday Life*. New York: Harper Collins, 1992.

Moravec, Hans. *Mind Children: The Future of Robot and Human Intelligence*. Cambridge, Mass.: Harvard University Press, 1988.

Munzel, G. Felicitas. *Kant's Conception of Moral Character*. Chicago: University of Chicago Press, 1999.

Murray, John Courtney. *We Hold These Truths*. New York: Sheed and Ward, 1960.

Murray, Patrick. *Reflections on Commercial Life*. New York: Routledge, 1997.

Myers, Steven Lee. "Whether to Bomb Is the Easy Part." *New York Times*, February 1, 1998.

Nagel, Thomas. "The Mind Wins." *The New York Review of Books*, March 4, 1993.

————. *Mortal Questions*. New York: Cambridge University Press, 1979.

————. *The View from Nowhere*. New York: Oxford University Press, 1986.

————. "War and Massacre." *International Ethics*. Edited by C. R. Beitz et al. Princeton, N.J.: Princeton University Press, 1985.

Needleman, Jacob. *Money and the Meaning of Life*. New York: Doubleday, 1991.

Nietzsche, Friedrich. *The Philosophy of Nietzsche*. Edited by Geoffrey Clive. New York: Mentor, 1965.

Noddings, Nel. *Caring: A Feminine Approach to Ethics and Moral Education*. Berkeley: University of California Press, 1978.

Norman, Richard. *Ethics of Killing and War*. New York: Cambridge University Press, 1995.

Norris, Christopher. *Uncritical Theory: Postmodernism, Intellectuals and the Gulf War*. Amherst: University of Massachussetts Press, 1992.

Nozick, Robert. *Anarchy, State and Utopia*. Oxford: Basil Blackwell, 1974.
———. *The Examined Life: Philosophical Meditations*. New York: Simon & Schuster, 1989.
Nussbaum, Martha, and Amartya Sen. *The Quality of Life*. Oxford: Clarendon Press, 1993.
Oliner, Samule, and Pearl M. Oliner. *The Altruistic Personality: Rescuers of Jews in Nazi Europe*. New York: Macmillan, 1988.
Olson, Eric T. *The Human Animal: Personal Identity without Psychology*. New York: Oxford University Press, 1997.
Ong, Walter, S.J. *Fighting for Life*. Ithaca, N.Y.: Cornell University Press, 1981.
———. *Hopkins, the Self and God*. Toronto: Toronto University Press, 1986.
Outka, Gene, and John Reeder, eds. *Prospects for a Common Morality*. Princeton: Princeton University Press, 1993.
Paglia, Camille. *Sex, Art and American Culture*. New York: Vintage, 1992.
Parfit, Derek. *Reasons and Persons*. Oxford: Clarendon Press, 1984.
Peck, M. Scott, M.D. *The Road Less Travelled*. New York: Simon & Schuster, 1978.
Penfield, Wilder. *The Mystery of the Mind*. Princeton, N.J.: Princeton University Press, 1975.
Percy, Walker. *Lost in the Cosmos*. New York: Washington Square Press, 1983.
Pernick, Martin S. *The Black Stork*. New York: Oxford University Press, 1996.
Pluhar, Evelyn. *Beyond Prejudice*. Durham, N.C.: Duke University Press, 1995.
Pojman, Louis, ed. *Life and Death: A Reader in Moral Problems*. Boston: Jones and Bartlett, 1993.
Porter, Jean. *The Recovery of Virtue*. Louisville, Ky.: Westminster Press, 1990.
Prejean, Helen, C.S.J. *Dead Man Walking: An Eyewitness Account of the Death Penalty in the United States*. New York: Random House, 1993.
Prunier, Gerard. *The Rwanda Crisis: History of a Genocide*. New York: Columbia University Press, 1995.
Puleo, Mev. *Mev Puleo: Witness to Life*. St. Louis: Samuel Cupples House and McNamee Gallery, 1997.
———. *The Struggle Is One*. Albany: State University of New York Press, 1994.
Rachels, James. *The End of Life: Euthanasia and Morality*. New York: Oxford University Press, 1987.
Ramsey, Paul. *The Just War: Force and Political Responsibility*. New York: Scribner, 1968.
Randall, Peter, ed. *Not Without Honour*. Johannesburg: Raven Press, 1982.
Rawls, John. *A Theory of Justice*. Cambridge, Mass.: Harvard University Press, 1971.
Reich, Walter. *Origins of Terrorism: Psychologies, Ideologies, Theologies, States of Mind*. New York: Cambridge University Press, 1990.
Restak, Richard, M.D. *The Mind*. New York: Bantam, 1988.

Ricoeur, Paul. *Freud and Philosophy: An Essay on Interpretation*. New Haven, Conn.: Yale University Press, 1970.

Rilke, Rainer Maria. *Letters to a Young Poet*. Translated by M. D. Herter Norton. New York: W. W. Norton, 1963.

Rorty, Amelie Oksenberg. *Mind in Action*. Boston: Beacon Press, 1988.

Rorty, Richard. *Consequences of Pragmatism*. Boston: Beacon Press, 1988.

———. *Contingency, Irony and Solidarity*. New York: Cambridge University Press, 1989.

———. *Philosophy and the Mirror of Nature*. Princeton, N.J.: Princeton University Press, 1979.

Rushkoff, Douglas. *Coercion: Why We Listen to What "They" Say*. New York: Penguin Putnam, 1999.

Ryle, Gilbert. *The Concept of Mind*. New York: Barnes & Noble, 1949.

Sacks, Oliver. *Awakenings*. New York: Harper Perennial, 1990.

———. *The Man Who Mistook His Wife for a Hat*. New York: Harper & Row, 1984.

Sartre, Jean-Paul. *Being and Nothingness*. Translated by Hazel Barnes. New York: Washington Square Press, 1966.

———. *The Transcendence of the Ego*. Translated by Forrest Williams and Robert Kirkpatrick. New York: Octagon Books, 1972.

Scheffler, Samuel, ed. *Consequentialism and Its Critics*. New York: Oxford University Press, 1988.

Schor, Juliet. *The Overspent American*. New York: Basic Books, 1998.

———. *The Overworked American*. New York: Basic Books, 1992.

Schrag, Calvin O. *Communicative Praxis and the Space of Subjectivity*. Bloomington: Indiana University Press, 1989.

———. *Experience and Being*. Evanston, Ill.: Northwestern University Press, 1969.

———. *The Resources of Rationality: A Response to the Post-Modern Challenge*. Bloomington: Indiana University Press, 1992.

———. *The Self after Postmodernity*. New Haven, Conn.: Yale University Press, 1997.

Schumacher, E .F. *Guide for the Perplexed*. New York: Harper & Row, 1977.

Searle, John. *The Rediscovery of the Mind*. Cambridge, Mass.: MIT Press, 1993.

———. *Mind, Language and Society*. New York: Basic Books, 1998.

Sebeok, Thomas, ed. *How Animals Communicate*. Bloomington: Indiana University Press, 1977.

———. *Speaking of Apes*. New York: Plenum: 1980.

Segaller, Stephen. *Invisible Armies: Terrorism into the 1990s*. New York: Harcourt Brance and Jovanovich, 1987.

Shames, Lawrence. *The Hunger for More: Searching for Values in an Age of Greed*. New York: Vintage, 1986.

Sherman, Nancy. *Making a Necessity of Virtue: Aristotle and Kant on Virtue*. New York: Cambridge University Press, 1997.

Shoumatoff, Alex. "Flight from Death." *The New Yorker*, June 20, 1994, 44–55.

Singer, Peter. *Animal Liberation*. New York: New York Review Press, 1990.

———. *Rethinking Life and Death*. New York: St. Martin's Press, 1995.

Skinner, B. F. *Beyond Freedom and Dignity*. New York: Bantam-Vintage, 1971.

———. *Science and Human Behavior*. New York: Macmillan, 1953.

Skorupski, John, ed. *The Cambridge Companion to Mill*. New York: Cambridge University Press, 1998.

Slater, Philip. *Wealth Addiction*. New York: Dutton, 1980.

Smart, J. J. C., and Bernard Williams, eds. *Utilitarianism: For and Against*. London: Cambridge University Press, 1973.

Steinbock, B., ed. *Killing and Letting Die*. Englewood Cliffs, N.J.: Prentice-Hall, 1980.

Steinman, Martin. "Rortyism." *Philosophy and Literature* 12 (1988): 27–47.

Stevenson, C. L. *Ethics and Language*. New Haven: Yale University Press, 1944.

———. *Facts and Values*. New Haven: Yale University Press, 1963.

Stivers, Richard. *The Culture of Cynicism*. Cambridge, Mass.: Blackwell, 1994.

Stout, Jeffrey. *Ethics After Babel: The Language of Morals and Their Discontents*. Boston: Beacon Press, 1988.

Stump, Eleonore. "Aquinas's Account of the Mechanisms of Intellective Cognition." *Revue Internationale de Philosophie*. February 1998.

———. "Non-Cartesian Substance Dualism and Materialism without Reductionism." *Faith and Philosophy* 12, no. 4 (October, 1995).

Sullivan, Roger. *An Introduction to Kant's Ethics*. New York: Cambridge, 1994.

———. *Kant's Moral Theory*. New York: Cambridge, 1989.

Sykes, Charles. *A Nation of Victims*. New York: St. Martin's Press, 1993.

Taylor, Charles. *The Ethics of Authenticity*. Cambridge, Mass.: Harvard University Press, 1991.

———. *Philosophical Papers 2: Human Agency and Language*. New York: Cambridge University Press, 1985.

———. *Sources of the Self: The Making of Modern Identity*. Cambridge, Mass.: Harvard University Press, 1989.

Terrace, Herbert. *Nim: A Chimpanzee Who Learned Sign Language*. New York: Alfred A. Knopf, 1979.

Thomas Aquinas. *On Being and Essence*, 2nd ed. Translated by Armand Maurer. Toronto: Pontifical Institute of Medieval Studies, 1968.

———. *Summa contra Gentiles*. Translated by Anton C. Pegis. Notre Dame, Ind.: University of Notre Dame Press, 1975.

———. *Summa Theologiae*. New York: Blackfriars/McGraw-Hill, 1963.

———. *Summa Theologiae: A Concise Translation*. Edited by Timothy McDermott Westminster, Md.: Christian Classics, 1989.

Thoreau, Henry David. *Walden and Civil Disobedience*. New York: Penguin, 1983 [1854].

Tolstoy, Leo. *The Death of Ivan Ilyitch and Other Stories*. Translated by Aylmer Maude. New York: New American Library, 1960.

Trefil, James. *Are We Unique? A Scientist Explores the Unparalleled Intelligence of the Human Mind*. New York: Wiley and Sons, 1997.

Turkle, Sherry. *The Second Self: Computers and the Human Spirit*. New York: Touchstone Books, 1984.

Twichell, James. *Lead Us Into Temptation*. New York: Columbia University Press, 1999.

de Unamuno, Miguel. *Tragic Sense of Life*. Princeton, N.J.: Princeton University Press, 1972.

Vanier, Jean. *Community and Growth: Our Pilgrimage Together*. New York: Paulist Press, 1979.

————. "Understanding our own Brokenness." In *Spiritual Journeys*. Edited by Stanislaus Kennedy. Dublin: Veritas, 1997.

Veatch, Henry. *Swimming Against the Current in Contemporary Philosophy*. Washington, D.C.: Catholic University of America Press, 1990.

Vining, Eileen P. G. et al. "Why Would You Remove Half a Brain? The Outcome of 58 Children After Hemispherectomy—The Johns Hopkins Experience: 1968 to 1996." *Pediatrics* 100, no. 2 (August 1997).

Walzer, Michael. *Just and Unjust Wars: A Moral Argument with Historical Illustrations*. New York: Basic Books, 1977.

Warren, Mary Ann. "Abortion." In *A Companion to Ethics*. Edited by Peter Singer. Cambridge: Blackwell, 1991.

————. "The Personhood Argument in Favor of Abortion." *The Monist* 57 (1973).

————. *Moral Status: Obligations to Persons and Other Living Things*. Oxford: Clarendon Press, 1997.

Washington State Medical Association, et al. *Pain Management and the Care of the Terminal Patient*. Seattle, Washington.

Weil, Simone. *Simone Weil*. Edited by Eric Springsted. Maryknoll, N.Y.: Orbis, 1988.

Weizenbaum, Joseph. *Computer Power and Human Reason: From Judgment to Calculation*. San Francisco: Freeman, 1976.

Wiesel, Elie. *Night*. New York: Avon Books, 1969.

Wilkes, Kathleen. *Real People: Personal Identity without Thought Experiments*. Oxford: Clarendon Press, 1988.

Williams, Bernard. *Ethics and the Limits of Philosophy*. Cambridge, Mass.: Harvard University Press, 1985.

————. *Making Sense of Humanity*. New York: Cambridge University Press, 1995.

————. *Problems of the Self.* New York: Cambridge University Press, 1976.

Williams, Patricia. *The Alchemy of Race and Rights.* Cambridge, Mass.: Harvard University Press, 1991.

Wilson, James Q. *The Moral Sense.* New York: Free Press, 1993.

Wittgenstein, Ludwig. *Letters to Russell, Keynes and Moore.* Ithaca, N.Y.: Cornell University Press, 1974.

Wolfe, Alan. *The Human Difference.* Berkeley: University of California Press, 1993.

Zahn, Gordon. *In Solitary Witness: The Life and Death of Franz Jägerstätter.* Collegeville, Minnesota: Liturgical Press, 1964.

Index

A2. *See* reflexive consciousness.

abortion debate, 125–32

academic world, depersonalized characteristics, 20–23, 205n6

actions as self-revelations, 42, 51–52, 69

Acts of Meaning (Bruner), 195n14

affirmation
of intrinsic values, 85–88, 107–08
as ownership, 60–62, 98–99

African Rights, 113

After Virtue (MacIntyre), 21, 161–62n2,
208n14

Allen, Woody, 110–12

*The Altruistic Personality: Rescuers of Jews in
Nazi Europe* (Oliner), 209n21

Amir, Yigal, 118

Amir Defense Line of Manhattan, 118

animal comparisons, 48, 49–50, 51, 68–69,
178–79n5, 179n6

Anscombe, Elizabeth, 208n14

a part/apart embodiment ambiguities, 37–
38

apartheid, Naude's actions, 104

Aquinas, Thomas, 1, 42–43, 48–49, 50, 51,
71, 75, 85–88, 93, 99, 106, 175n16,
176n21, 187–89n11

Aristotle, 44, 51

assisted suicide. *See* euthanasia.

authenticity ideal (Taylor's discussion),
191–93n9

autonomy argument in abortion, 128

autonomy/liberty in moral choice, 92–93

avoidance/yearning dilemma, 14–17

awareness experiments, 45, 177n24

awareness of awareness. *See* reflexive
consciousness.

Baillie, James, 171–72n4

Bauby, Jean-Dominque, 154

Beauchamp, Tom L., 198n13

Becker, Ernest, 210–11n30

Belk, Russell, 144–45

Bellah, Robert, 168n13

Benetton advertising, 145

Benhabib, Seyla, 184–85n5

Bennis, Warren, 204–05n5

Bernstein, Richard, 23, 161–63n2

Bettelheim, Bruno, 13

*Beyond Prejudice: The Moral Significance of
Human and Nonhuman Animals* (Pluhar),
68–69

birth argument of personhood,
127–28

Black, Sir Douglas, 196–97n5

The Black Stork (movie), 136–37

body. *See* embodiment.

Boethius, 64, 65

bombing logic, 115–18

Bono (rock star), 144, 146

brain argument of personhood, 127

*Bright Air, Brilliant Fire: On the Matter of the
Mind* (Edelman), 164–65n4

Brink, David, 186–87n8

Brothers Karamazov (Dostoyevsky), 138,
150–51

Bruner, Jerome, 195n14

Buber, Martin, 35

Callahan, Daniel, 149, 209n19

Callahan, Joseph, 184n4

Camus, Albert, 14–15, 109–10,
196n19

Can't We Make Moral Judgements
(Midgley), 191n7

capital punishment, 104–05, 125

career nature of personhood, 62–64,
181–82n18

Carney, Guadalupe, 19

Cartesian ego, 28, 30

Cassidy, Sheila, 155–56